FROM THE INSIDE OUT

FROM THE INSIDE OUT

An Artists' Expression Through Healing
From Traumatic Brain Injury

Cara Mayo

For Jared and Oren Gruber, always in my heart

Published By The Creative Short Book Writers Project
Wayne Drumheller, Editor and Founder
Publishing and Printing Platform: Createspace
Book and Cover Design by Jared Gruber and Writing As Art & Publishing
Distribution in the USA by Cara Mayo email: brudewolfe@yahoo.com and www.Amazon.com.

ISBN-13: 978:1721257737
ISBN-10: 172125773X

From The Inside Out: An Artist' Expression Through Healing From Traumatic Brain Injury is copyrighted and published by Cara Mayo, 2018 All Rights Reserved. All Art, illustrations, writings and notes are created and ® registered by the author, unless otherwise ascribed to another noted writer. The quotes found in this book are, to best of my ability, what I heard, felt, believed and remembered when they were spoken, read or inferred to me. This book cannot be reproduced or copied in any part without the expressed permission of the author. It is made possible, in part, by a one-time gift-in-kind sponsorship of time, book design, and editing assistance from the Creative Short Book Writers Project. Since 2010, the project has been a self-funded and sustainable project by the author. No part of this book may be reproduced or transmitted in any form or by any means, electronic or mechanical, including photocopying, recording or by any information storage and retrieval system without the expressed permission of the author, except for brief quotations embodied in articles or otherwise specified.

FROM THE INSIDE OUT

CONTENTS

Introduction, Page 3

Chapter I, Page 4
TBI-1, Page 8
TBI-2, Page 10
TBI-3, Page 13

Paintings

Painting 1, I'm Melting. Page 16
Painting 2, Going To Bits, Page 20
Painting 3, All of This And More, Page 24
Painting 4, A Broken Path, Page 28
Painting 5, Somewhere Beats A Heart, Page 32
Painting 6, Somewhere There Is Light, Page 36
Painting 7, Tilt, Page 40
Painting 8, Wings Of Hope, Page 46
Painting 9, Looking For Stillness, Page 50
Painting 10, Clearing, Page 54
Painting 11, From The Inside Out, Page 60
Painting 12, Tides Of Change, Page 64
Chapter II, Page 68
Chapter III, Page 71
Acknowledgements, Page 71
About The Paintings, Page 72

My Gallery

Before the Accident 2004, Page 73
Painting from 2005-2015, Page 74
Artwork from 2016-2018, Page 75

INTRODUCTION

The facts of my traumatic brain injury (TBI) and care are: Aug. 1, 2004 head injury with slight gash on right temple. Loss of awareness for one to three hours. Broken clavicle and rib with very bruised upper right side. Damaged rotator cuff, left shoulder.

I got immediate attention for the broken bones but waited one month to see a neurologist. The hospital I was taken to following the accident didn't do an MRI or CAT Scan, nor did the neurologist suggest them. Fortunately, even in my brain-fogged state, I knew I had to move home in order to survive. Six months after the accident I saw a neurologist in the Syracuse, N.Y. area. He had the MRI and CAT Scan done. The MRI showed slight damage to the back of my brain. The neurologist recommended that I see a neuropsychologist for testing and symptom management.

A nurse friend of mine brought me to a meeting with a doctor from University Hospital's head trauma unit. I spoke with the doctor and after the meeting called the hospital as he suggested. It was the best thing that I did for my recovery. Starting with my initial phone call, all of the people I talked to in the head trauma unit were wonderful working with me. People who see a large number of head trauma patients recognize and respond to them in ways that provide a lifeline through the myriad challenges. It took eight months for me to get to University Hospital. Some of the suffering that I lived with for eight months was dispelled in one day. I wonder how life would have been if I had gotten attention of this kind sooner.

I met with a neuro-ophthalmologist in Syracuse, New York and learned that a large number of concussion patients, regardless of age, suffer from dry eye. The constant, intense, behind-the-eyes headache the drugs couldn't touch was gone in two days after I started using over-the-counter eye drops for dry eye. My visual acuity was back to normal, having gotten much worse from dry eye. I still had significant symptoms with my vision and continue to work with these symptoms.

In the years after my accident, I felt compelled to document my experiences through paintings, prose, and stories. I am still healing, thankfully. And I still believe that I will be better than normal eventually. Each day I learn more and look for alternative ways to move through life. At this time normal life is filled with challenges. I have days when I learn more and look for a new way of learning because of necessity. Now I realize that this practice is a more truthful, joyful, courageous experience that I will endeavor to continue regardless of where I am with healing.

This ultimately broader view and support system allows me to flow with life when previously I was unable to accept life on such a grand scale. Rather than view the TBI as limiting, it has become a way-shower for greater wholeness. In order to have the courage to reach out for another paradigm, a strong support is a necessity for me. It is useful for personal journeying and to shield from negative labels, responses and assumptions from interior and exterior sources.

I suggest that you read this account with the interest of living in a creative way rather than as a plan for TBI treatment. Then it will remain in the spirit in which it was lived and is intended as a humble path uniquely mine but similar in many ways to the path that each one of us walks every day.

Note: This book was written in stages. Stage 1 was paintings, prose and drawings in 2006, introduction and painting explanations in 2007, stories and corrections in 2018.

Chapter 1

At my first meeting with Dr. Landes, my psychologist at University Hospital, he said to me that every concussion patient who walked into his office felt that they should be able to resume their life as it was prior to the concussion. The inability to return to their previous life often left them feeling guilty, disbelieving, hopeless, fearful and frustrated. I had these feelings regularly for almost three years after the accident.

The biggest hurdle is internal compared to outside challenges. When well-meaning family and friends had post-concussion expectations or made comments about the frequency of my memory lapses and sensitivities it would throw me into a deeper pit of self-destructive mental chatter. During a visit with Dr. Landes I relayed a situation to him. His brief comment about close family being in denial was another milestone toward healing. I learned to stop the set up to failure and instead tune into what I could do. Then I learned to tell people what I could do. Eventually I felt good about what I accomplished regardless of how small it was. And I was released from the denial, having given it back to its originator.

My first day at University Hospital gave me tools and hope. I continued to get wonderful care from my team through physical, occupational, and psychological therapy and neuro-ophthalmologist visits, along with a nurse practitioner in the wings. Eventually I had neuropsychology testing. In October 2004 I started chiropractic care that I continued to receive until 2006. It was very helpful. I received weekly "One Brain" and "Touch for Health" therapy from a dear friend. I tried other alternative-healing modalities after doing research about them or based on suggestions by friends. It became evident to me that I had to be careful about how I healed. The stress of traveling to an appointment could negate any healing.

Time after time I returned to simple, spontaneous choices. Listening to the sounds of nature for countless days when I couldn't open my eyes. (By May 2005 I was able to use my eyes for three hours without intense pain.) Feeling the sun and wind on my body, enjoying the feeling of petting an animal, touching a wool sweater or silk, imagining the feeling of colors or the taste of sounds and colors—anything that filled me with richness helped. Visual and hearing sensitivities precipitated the desire for quiet and dark.

The stress of coping with the sound of a TV in another room became almost unbearable and burned brain energy quickly, rendering me useless for triple the amount of TV time. My nights were filled with interruptions and sleeplessness until January 2007 when I started having nights that I slept through until 6:00 a.m. Sleeping wasn't really a time of rest and healing. The hours spent listening to nature stopped the mental chatter and gave me the quiet, relaxing, healing time that I needed. I was very aware of my brain clock ticking away and lived with the fear that one stressful moment could incapacitate me.

On the days when I felt my brain was "seeing" (technically my eyes were fine), I would drive. At first it was for short trips and well-traveled routes. I had a bag with overnight things in case I didn't feel capable of driving home after visiting a friend. Slowly I stretched my muscles in different directions, for the most part at my own pace. I am still doing that. Today I have more knowledge and confidence but the unknown still looms. I have and still put myself into challenging situations and make mistakes. I get frightened about mistakes but look in other directions for support and answers rather than sitting in fear. I have transferred my creativity and intuition to everyday living. It took me a while to realize that what I thought of as brain healing was really a better-tuned intuitive sense.

Two days after the accident I returned to my apartment. Fortunately my dear friend Ann and her husband Bill, along with my son Oren and his wife at the time, alternated caring for me. I would have stayed in bed—not moving, eating or doing anything—if I was left alone. I was in pain constantly, mentally lost. I existed in a state of thick cotton pain that wound through me and wrapped around me, and nothing occurred to me. Everything was incredibly difficult. I only knew that something was really wrong. In the early days I looked injured and people responded accordingly.

Later, when I looked more normal, things became more difficult. I don't know how I first realized that something was wrong. Perhaps it was the constant pain or the recognition that I was miles away when trying to communicate or understand. Somehow I knew that life changed. People told me things but I didn't understand. It was as if speech bubbles were coming out of their mouths. It was hard to translate what they were saying to me, to make it mine. It was through the slow process of existence and being around normal life in small doses that growth happened. In the first month after the accident, somehow it came to mind that I would choose how to enrich my brain. As a child we don't have choices. We are subject to the circumstances we grow up in. I decided to actively choose.

A fortnight before the accident I had returned from a trip to Ireland. We traveled to two very old sacred sites and I saw magnificent trees. It would take me a full day to try to recollect one tree. I sat on the sofa all day and tried to remember one tree, the feeling and details of that tree. Each day a different tree. I rarely remembered what the tree actually looked like but I could get a sense of it. I did my first watercolor painting of a tree in September 2004. The challenge of using a three-inch by five-inch paper was all that I could manage and I had to paint using my non-dominant hand. Eventually I did 12 small paintings of trees.

Whenever I realized that my thoughts were chaotic I would return to visualizing a tree. That was my first step. During that time I remember telling my daughter-in-law, "I don't know who I am, where I am or where I am going. Whatever you see or feel from me has nothing to do with you, only with me. I will speak up if I need something, or if I am bothered please do your own thing and don't worry."

Now I realize this is still true for my life today. Some of the early lessons brought me to a truer understanding of how to live a contented life. I firmly held on to the idea that I needed to spend as much time as possible in a positive state. I refused to accept the looks or words that reflected "poor you" and the limitations that this was a life setback. Instead I went back to my very vivid memory just before and during the accident.

It was the wonderful contentment I had riding in the car on a nice sunny day with joyful expectations for a lovely evening. Then an even stronger memory enveloped me. I was somewhere floating in this very dark, black, warm place. I had never seen such deep blackness and yet I felt a sense of joy, love, freedom and being-ness that expanded to an unending vastness. A feeling of fertility and expectancy surrounded and filled me. I tried to find my body but I couldn't find it. I did sense the brightness of my consciousness. In the far distance I saw gentle lapping waves in this vast, dark, rich sea with pinpricks of different colored lights that took on a vibrant gemstone quality. It was beautiful watching the lights bob on the waves.

When I realized the beautiful bobbing lights were souls I began to look for my colored light. At that instant out of the blackness arose a silhouette of my mother and aunt sitting on a park bench. They were kicking their feet like children do in a happy, carefree way. I started to look beyond my mother and aunt to a breathtaking skyscape. At that moment mom said to me, "Cara, everything will be just fine."

And then I was in the emergency outpatient room seeing the nurse in front of me. I believe there was a one- to three-hour gap in my conscious memory. My friend told me she asked the ambulance to take me to a hospital with a good head trauma unit. She said that after the Ford Explorer SUV hit her car I sat completely still with my eyes open, not moving. When she talked to me I didn't respond and she was afraid that I was dead. It took some time before I moved and more time before I moved and finally responded to her. The EMTs had to go through the driver-side door to get me out and on a stretcher. The SUV hit just behind the passenger door and totaled the car. I knew that I was tossed around even with the seatbelt on. My left shoulder was bruised and my right temple also. I had a broken clavicle and rib.

The experience I had seeing my recently deceased mother and aunt is called a near-death experience (NDE). There are books and an organization called the International Association for Near Death Studies (IANDS) that can give more information on NDEs. While there may be controversy on this subject, from personal experience I know NDEs exist. The experience I had filled me with love, hope and a more universal outlook. It was the cornerstone for my recovery.

The moment I became conscious I had a vivid memory of the NDE. I knew without a doubt that I would be just fine. I didn't have worries about permanent mental or physical loss. When I became discouraged, angry, hopeless or pain-filled I would remember what my mother said to me during the NDE. When I attended my first TBI support group meeting years later I listened to the stories from other people. While I had lived through many of the same symptoms, I didn't have the fear.

I still wonder how to ease the fears of concussion patients. When the body is in a stress mode it isn't healing and growing. Fear prevents healing. I was not aware of this at the time. I did know that chaotic thoughts and feelings needed to be replaced by positive ones.

It took some time to catch on and then to stop the flow of fear before I could reseed with positive messages. I had a deep memory of the experience with my mother and aunt and I could wrap myself in that feeling of wholeness, oneness and love. Very simply I had the NDE to support me. And I collected other information along the way to further support my positive growth. The NDE provided me with the knowledge to disagree with or ignore what other people said and helped show me the direction to look for positive growth.

It took creativity to find my way. I was open to and available for anything that would support healing. I knew I was going to recover and I was willing to look for support no matter how small. Because my journey was long and hard I tried to do no harm to others. There were many times when my behavior felt hurtful or offensive to other people. I tried my best. I remember hearing someone tell me that I should have told them about my symptoms and what I was going through.

It didn't occur to me at the time to talk about my experience and I didn't have the words to use. In fact I worked very hard to not talk about how I was feeling. I am still amazed at the amount of resistance close family and friends had to my symptoms.

In my most challenging times I had to steer through a new inner world while trying to cope with uneducated family and friends. They often held me to high standards and took me to task for not complying. In this way I learned that usually life is all about each person's world. The most unconditional and loving people that I have met are near-death experiencers. I have valued the times at meetings when I was cared for just as I was. Those times were the closest to the actual NDE I felt while living in a conscious state.

Most experiencers know how precious every sentient being is, how precious and wonderful life is. There is also the lack of fear of death. Most experiencers didn't want to return from their NDE; I didn't. We know where we will go when physical life ceases. It represents a transition to joy, not fear.

The paintings in this book and the writings that go with them came about when I was far enough from the original experience and yet not out of it. On one hand I didn't want to get engulfed and on the other I wanted to be fresh with it. There was no planning, only the feeling that came suggesting the time was near when I would re-enter the journey. The pattern of painting and writing is one I have used most of my adult life. It is a way for me to digest and intimately touch.

I have done plein air painting and painted from my photos in the studio. My journaling solidified when I seriously studied various religions and meditative techniques. The process of painting and journaling was comfortable for me but the subject matter wasn't. I have learned a degree of objectivity and watchfulness. Therefore each painting and description took a very short amount of time. I found a series of three paintings, created quickly with acrylic paint and then written about in order, to be the desired pattern. Then the colored pencil drawings with an explanation came next.

Contrary to my usual need to paint only in daylight, these paintings happened at night when it was dark outside and quiet. I didn't need light to see what I was painting. It was a process of emptying out and trying to do so in the cleanest, quickest most truthful manner. After each series I made copies and brought them to show Dr. Landes. This is my first look at them (2007) since they were created. It is with mixed feelings that I re-enter the experience.

TBI Story 1

There were experiences that arose during recovery from the traumatic brain injury (TBI). I was always stunned and frightened when they occurred. When I first saw a cartoon bubble with squiggles in it coming from a person's mouth, and had no idea what the person was saying, it was instant panic. My brain had crashed, which meant it would only get worse (reset took a few days). Fear loomed about what might happen next as more brain services went offline. Often people would repeat what they said and I would see the same squiggles in a cloud coming from their mouth with more insistence for response. The best I could do was to shrug or say "oh" or find another nonresponse, wave, smile and walk away acutely mindful of holding together what was still functioning so I wouldn't trip, step into traffic or bump into someone.

If I was walking I would find a private place to sit, close my eyes and attempt to calm down while going over where I was and how I would get home. When I had driven I would find my car and sit in it while I collected my remaining energy to focus on where I was, the route home and how I could manage the trip. I traveled with an overnight bag in my car so I could spend the night at a friend's house if I felt unsafe to drive. Friends' houses were part of the calibration process as I monitored myself and my ability to focus while attempting to use as little energy and brainpower as possible. They were high-stress times, and for adrenal glands stuck in constant fatigue it was horrendous.

Usually when I had to go to appointments at University Hospital, the cartoon bubbles would appear. It was intensely stressful to drive on an interstate highway and find my way through Syracuse, N.Y. to the hospital's parking garage. I always wrote in big letters and short notations the exit and streets to take. Unfortunately after about four notations my brain couldn't process and I had to maneuver by intuition. Often I would pull over to rest my eyes and collect myself only to realize my destination was across the street or in front of me. I traveled this way starting in 2005—a year after the TBI, when I began driving again—and it continues to this day. I have graduated to two more notations now.

Having an appointment at the hospital meant I had to park in a parking garage. Definitely an upsetting prospect when my brain didn't function well. I would wait on the ground level until a car left a parking spot because I couldn't manage going up or down ramps. The ramps didn't make visual sense to me. Therefore I gave myself two hours to get to an appointment when the actual total time would have been 35 minutes. Once I got a parking space I had to collect myself and refer to the map I had drawn to walk to and maneuver in the hospital. The hospital had fluorescent lights, a death knell for my eyes and brain.

With oversensitivity, anything visual, sounds, smells and other people's energy make for a landmine of overwhelm. I have always been overly sensitive to other people's feelings—knowing and feeling more than I wanted to. I have always felt the child near-death experience (NDE), at four years old, was the starting point. The adult NDE during the accident and resulting TBI increased my sensitivities. I recoiled from layers of emotions, piled on over the years, at the hospital. Like a worn carpet the embedded information could bring me to my knees. I had to use valuable brain energy to block the emotions under my feet and above and around me, while shielding from the lights and the people and all other information bombarding my senses.

I was told with TBI the part of the brain that buffers information is damaged. The times when we are at a public place talking to people, our brain filters out the activity and noises around us so we can focus on what is happening in front of us. That is the buffer at work. Without the buffer everything happening is just as insistent for our attention as what is in front of us. Every noise, sight, smell has to be noticed and manually turned down, only to repeat the process a few seconds later.

Leakage of brain energy brought confusion, dizziness, nausea and overwhelm with more brain services shutting down. Hospital appointments always created more brain fatigue from the simple questions asked to the physical rehabilitation and reading and math tests or psychology tests. I was assigned a team of five practitioners at University Hospital for my recovery, with a neuro-ophthalmologist added on. The neuro-ophthalmologist was at an offsite location with a wonderful big parking lot behind the building. After a lengthy exam I was told I had dry eye, which is a lack of lubrication from a nonfunctioning or poorly functioning tear duct and is very common with head trauma. The symptoms of dry eye include loss of visual acuity and behind-the-eye headaches. Since the accident I constantly had headaches of this kind of varying intensity that drugs didn't help. The over-the-counter eye drops for dry eye were a miracle for me. The constant headaches slowly relented. The neuro-ophthalmologist told me that over time my eyes might begin to produce tears again. After a number of years I didn't need the eye drops.

I was also told that my eyes were stuck in a constant action of moving in and out and side to side, much like a camera lens trying to focus. The doctor was taken aback that I was driving and suggested it wasn't a good idea, that my depth perception would be especially difficult. I explained there was no other way for me to get to appointments. My family and friends were working and buses weren't available. During the entire recovery time I went to all of my appointments alone, with the exception of my initial visits to a neurologist and to a sports doctor for rotator cuff damage and a broken collar bone and rib.

The neuro-ophthalmologist suggested I try glasses with prisms to help my eyes focus better. Trying to walk in a hallway with prism glasses created dizziness and nausea. It was decided I would get dark, thick frames for my glasses to help my eyes focus in front of me. The constant eye movement might decrease as my brain healed. This did happen slowly. About one-and-a-half years after the accident the constant dizziness and nausea stopped, although I still had bouts of that. Before using the dry-eye drops I had about two hours a day where I could open my eyes without intense headaches. Even with the eye drops, reading two lines of print was the most I could manage before a headache arose. It was a long, slow process.

TBI Story 2

When I returned from the hospital, a dear friend of mine, my daughter-in-law at the time and my son took turns taking care of me. I wasn't able to sleep. The constant pain and mental turmoil coupled with hypervigilance kept me awake. I existed somewhere and was acutely aware that my body was a shell for my consciousness. When my caregivers brought me to the table to eat, that's when I ate. It never occurred to me to eat. Energy usage was the first major lesson my body and brain taught me. In the beginning I was frozen in pain and shock. The effort and energy I needed to get up and move around often exceeded the energy that was available to me.

The hospital also gave me a prescription for pain medicine. The first night home I took the medication and I felt so terrible that I refused to take any again. The only meds I took were over-the-counter headache relief, and when that didn't work I stopped taking anything. One year after the accident the nurse practitioner I was seeing prescribed Ritalin, half of the smallest dose available. I tried it for three days and stopped. Even though my brain wasn't functioning I knew that I needed to feel and know what was going on with my brain and body. Medication for me only scrambled the information. I also knew that I needed to embrace the pain, to learn what it was teaching me. I couldn't run from the pain or push it away; that took too much effort and revisited me later in other ways.

The constant memory that comforted and supported me, from the moment I woke up in the emergency room, throughout recovery and to this day, was the near-death experience (NDE) I had during the accident. The NDE arose from the blackness—a vivid, loving, imprint on my consciousness that flowed in and was more real than anything my physical senses could experience. I still don't have words for the intensity of the experience. The supreme feeling during the NDE was Oneness. The experience brought me to a knowingness of the connection of my consciousness with the vastness beyond. I went to a point of dissolution, bathing in the vastness of the universe and feeling a sense of Oneness and intense freedom. I would have gratefully continued the process but my deceased mother called me back.

It was the second-most disappointing experience I can remember. The first was a child NDE when I had to return.

This physical existence is a shadow of the intensity I felt during the NDE. The Oneness, love, compassion and joy that surrounded and filled my consciousness eclipsed the limitations of living from my body. My brain wasn't working, but when something arose through my body to move me in a particular direction I accepted that it was the best choice for me. I saw that every sentient being was surrounded by love and compassion. Their awareness of and openness to this limitless love is the deciding factor. (Know that we are all surrounded by love at all times and can be filled with this love if we allow it.) When being here feels challenging I turn inside to my connection to Spirit and do what is in front of me: washing dishes, folding towels etc. Oneness is about being a conduit for Spirit.

While I didn't understand the suffering I was experiencing, embracing it was a pathway to Spirit and the only thing that worked for me.

It is amusing to watch myself paint, whether landscape, portrait or abstract, and let the process continue beyond the initial voice to be expressed. I always end up painting dissolution, through the deep, dark, star-filled Universe into the blackness of the Void, something that can never be expressed. Painting for me is about stopping the process at a time when it needs to end and seeing what is emerging. There is information for me to embrace visually before I continue the process or put the painting aside. These expressions are a way to watch the ripples of Spirit move through me to the canvas while the mental mind pauses. Beyond words, embracing the process so that it becomes part of my being-ness, holding a space for the voice of this experience to move through me, I am filled with gratitude.

A month after the accident I painted 10 trees using watercolors. They were trees I saw in Ireland three months prior to the accident. The paintings depicted the energy impression of each tree, not the actual tree. The wonder of those trees imprinted themselves on me as they became a lifeline for the initial steps of my recovery. In the many days of partial existence a tree connection would occur, unfolding the energy of the tree and the land it grew from. The land and trees were sacred places for me. I would spend all day with that one tree, frozen on the couch in inactivity. It was all that I had, all that I could do.

Two years later I was working on a painting from a photo I had taken. I used the grid system, drawing pencil lines on the canvas and the photo so I could more accurately paint the subject. Now, this entire exercise was a great deal of effort and pain for me. To even focus on a ruler and draw lines was a great challenge. I suddenly realized while painting that I had transferred the photo information from one square into the wrong square on my painting. The subject was ruins of an architectural structure so correct placement was important. And then I noticed what I had just repainted was incorrect and I fixed the square again, finally causing me to step back and look at the entire painting. Everything was wrong. When I stepped away from the canvas to look again, I saw all of the squares shift. For the next few minutes I changed where I was standing and watched the squares move. That was when I really realized my eye/brain connection was really screwed up. The words from the neuro-ophthalmologist sunk in.

At that point I put a mark on the floor showing exactly where I had to stand to work on the painting. Slowly the squares were repainted until I had a completed piece. I never told anyone about this at the time and only shared this experience a few times. It was just how life was at the time. I was very determined to return to who I was before the accident and didn't have the energy or mental space to truly explore what happened. I learned that if I wanted to paint I had to stay in the exact same place during the process. So many things were closed to me (biking, swimming, running, long walks, reading, movies, TV, computers etc.) that I had to hang on to something from my previous life in whatever way I could. And with the intense eye/brain focus it usually took a few days of sitting and doing nothing to put the stuffing back. I was still at the point where the sound from TV or music put me into overwhelmed, and I had to find a way to escape the torture.

Fast-forward 14 years later, I almost never watch a movie (maybe one per year) and I don't own a TV or use a computer unless I absolutely have to. My cellphone provides access to the internet, which I can use for short time periods to spread out the eye strain. Fortunately as each year passes I am increasing the time I can use my cellphone at one sitting. This is a long way from the days of being proficient in Photoshop.

To maximize my energy usage I walked away from loud noises, people sending out strong energy (especially negative), confusing visual information and the sense of touch.

There were times when positive subjects would change into negative spaces, like the time a friend was driving and the toll booth lane looked solid but the toll booth didn't. Until six years ago, while driving occasionally, the street information I was driving through would switch to visual cues from another city I had visited. I learned to carefully pull over and wade through the information until I got the visual cues for the current city, not as straightforward a process as you would expect. There was still a part of me that watched my actions. If I felt uncertain in any way at any time, I wouldn't go out or I would turn around and go home. I gave myself time to collect my energy and organize myself before setting off. Traveling from one safe landmark to another was the way I chose my routes. Any blips caused my already stressed adrenal glands to escalate. I had to find ways to decrease stress in order to continue and not become frozen. Mantras helped bypass the hypervigilant fear messages and allowed my intuition to operate. It was amazing to feel the flow of a route that asserted itself.

In 2010 I had to drive to a series of doctor appointments in Annapolis, Maryland from my apartment in Northern Virginia. At that time there was construction on a part of 395 North that connected the highway to Route 50/301. You had to exit 395 and take an auxiliary road to rejoin 395 again.

I meticulously wrote directions for traveling on 395 and another route through Washington, D.C. to Route 50. Mass transit wasn't available to my destination. I planned the first trip to avoid the confusion of driving through D.C. and traveling on 395 but it didn't work that way. I ended up in D.C. driving around lost with nowhere to pull over, frantically looking at my notes and maps while at a stoplight. When my brain could no longer read and I was getting tunnel vision, I kept repeating to myself the name of the street that would take me to Route 50 out of D.C. and toward Annapolis. I threw the papers on the floor and drove by intuition, finding the street shortly after and getting to my destination safely. That trip included a three-hour window for travel. The return trip that day was faster because I surrendered to the drive through D.C. rather than overriding my intuition and taking 395.

On another trip I took the wrong exit and was at a stoplight in a rough part of D.C. when police cars with sirens swarmed toward a street adjacent to the one I was on. People were running toward the commotion and I was looking for a way out. I made a U-turn in the middle of the street before oncoming traffic could move and found my way back to the interstate highway. I would love to say I finally became proficient on that route but I didn't. It was a very happy time when I no longer needed to make that trip.

TBI Story 3

Familiar surroundings, family and friends are all very important to me. They were my only touchstone with the life that I left and with the life that I hoped to put together.

In 2015 I worked with Dr. Mark Gordon of Millennium Health Centers. He prescribed regular blood draws to find out what glands were functioning. My cortisol level in 2015, 11 years after the accident, was 25.6 ug/dl, which is considered high. (Normal is 15 ug/dl.) I was on my way to adrenal shutdown. My baseline adrenal functioning was stuck on high alert all of the time. Think about the way you feel hearing upsetting news, having an argument or driving in traffic. Jump that mind/body response higher and hold it there. That was my baseline stress level. The scope of upsetting occurrences increased because I didn't have the ability to sort through what was potentially harmful and what wasn't. In hypervigilance everything created a ripple. Two people having a quiet disagreement in a room near my bedroom would jolt me wide awake from sleep and fill me with trepidation.

I lived and drove in Arlington from 2007 through 2016. With all of the traffic, people and constant noise, I was getting worse. My last-ditch decision in 2016 to move to the country near a small, quiet town was all I could think to do. Before moving there, I had never lived in the country, I knew only one acquaintance who lived 13 miles from the town and I had spent all of one hour visiting the town. After I moved there, I finally started sleeping. I got to a place where driving around and getting lost was upsetting but doable because there was little traffic. For me, living in a small town is helping me heal. I miss so many things about living in Arlington, especially family, but I couldn't exist there.

Essential oils from Young Living (therapeutic-grade quality) have been a constant companion in my recovery since my first Raindrop treatment in 2005. Nine oils are put along the spine. The treatment helped awaken my brain. The olfactory part of the brain is one of the oldest areas. Each oil helped stimulate my brain in different ways. I never left the house without them and still travel with some in my purse.

When I started cooking for myself in 2005 I began using organic foods and dropped sugar, flour, dairy, caffeine and alcohol. I eat this way today. When I go out and have foods I normally don't eat, I notice that my brain and body don't function as well. Because my primary concern is supporting my brain, I'm pretty conscientious about how I eat. A water purification system is important as well.

FROM THE INSIDE OUT

In 2015 I read a book called *Medical Medium* (copyright 2015) by Anthony William. At age four, Anthony heard a divine voice telling him when someone was ill. He reads people's health conditions and tells them how to recover. His journey to becoming a medical medium is fascinating. The suggestions he had for healing adrenal fatigue helped me tremendously. Anthony said that when the brain runs out of useful fuel, the adrenals kick in to keep the brain functioning. Having a small, healthy snack combination every 90 minutes gives the brain a steady fuel source and lets the adrenals rest. I instantly felt relieved and more relaxed. Celery, apple, carrots, avocado and a date or orange went with me every day. I used the supplements and ate the foods Anthony suggested. Shortly after I started this protocol I worked with Dr. Gordon and took the supplements he prescribed. Concurrently I started doing sessions on a Ceragem chi bed twice a week. You lie down on the chi bed and small golf-ball-size pieces of jade are heated with far-infrared light; they then move along your spine, stimulating acupressure points. I'd been existing in a frozen body for 11 years. The chi bed stimulated my body and helped me slowly unfold. After I moved in 2016 I didn't have access to the chi bed. Eight months after I moved, my mind and body functioning deteriorated noticeably. I purchased a chi bed and it was a great decision.

Walking, exercising, tai chi, chi gong, Pilates and yoga are all very helpful to do whenever you can. I learned not to push myself but to let the exercise arise when my body and brain felt energized and less stressed. Exercise is stress. Tai chi or chi gong are more flowing, so perhaps they would be easier for some people to do. I find allowing my body to move in a flowing state helps me awaken and doesn't tax my mind to remember or copy what comes next.

I am aware that my issues related to TBI have been very hard for my family and friends. Some people have dropped off along the way. I had trouble living with myself and still do, so it is no surprise that others find me challenging. What I am noticing since 2016, as I heal I step out a little bit more and inhabit this physical body with more inner light. It is a process, and I am better this year than I was last year. That spark of connection with Spirit that we all have is the go-to place for continual support. In the beginning the knowingness of love and compassion from the NDE carried me through.

Family and friends can help a TBI person feel they are in a sacred space; it could be in nature sitting near a special tree regularly, spending time with a pet, watching birds on a bird feeder or looking at the mountains. If that isn't possible, pictures or a poster on the wall of a peaceful place can be used. Doing your best to be with the person in a calm, loving way supports healing. When someone around me was frustrated or angry, I knew it and took it on as my having created more stress for that person. For this entire recovery I have been aware of and concerned about being a burden to others, even people I don't know well. It was this underlying feeling of being a burden that pushed me to drive when I wasn't ready, to do without many things and to make myself small. The only thing I could hold on to was to do no harm to others. I am not suggesting there is never a disagreement with someone else; I'm saying be mindful about your choices.

Starting the day with gratitude and reviewing things to be grateful for during the hard times is very helpful. What we put out we get back. If you want to live a more joyful life, put out more joy—even if it means finding joy watching birds or a flower or the rain. We live in the small things; they add up. I spend a lot of time sending compassion and love to people, animals and the earth. Let more and more of my thoughts create waves of positive energy. That is my goal.

I often wonder about the superpowers I told Dr. Landes I was watching for. Maybe a superpower is knowing from the ground up that Spirit fills me and surrounds me with love and compassion always. And knowing this walk on earth is sacred and that I choose moment to moment how to do it. Choosing gratitude and compassion as much as I can and supporting Oneness is my best contribution.

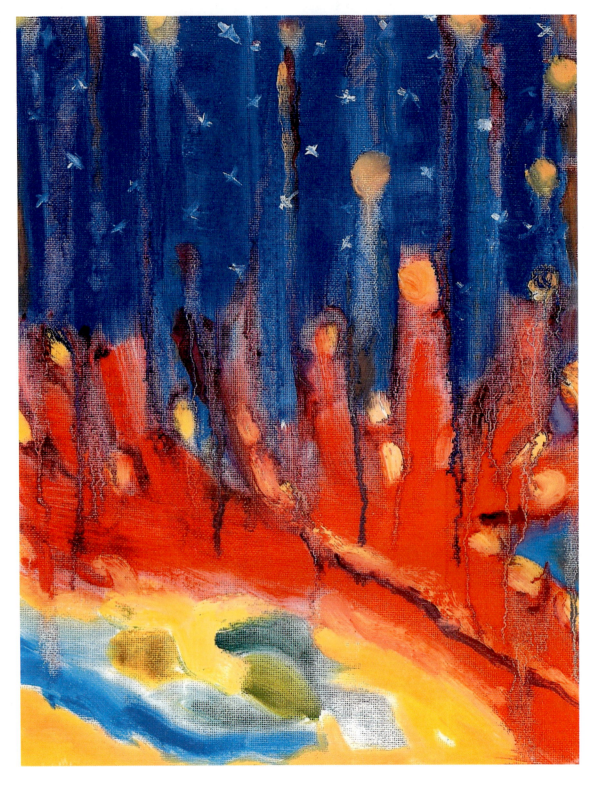

Painting 1 "I'm Melting"

Prose Painting 1 I'm Melting

I am lost in the stars. Things are melting. I see trees and dark night with millions of white twinkling stars.

I am afraid to look down.

Afraid that I will see nothing or only something partially there and it will engulf me.

I don't want to be lost but all I have is to gaze upward. Whatever reaches me hear are echoes. Echoes that bounce from trees and are lost in the icy dark sky.

Sometimes I feel a warm hand down there trying to reach me.

It is red and small, just like my hand. I think it will feel worse to try to grasp that hand and slip because our hands are red and wet.

I don't want to go down there.

Sometimes my feet sink into sponge and I am afraid that I will be lost, I will crumble.

I am holding this tree for support or I will be totally lost.

Sometimes a drop splashes on me. A drop from above. Am I am melting, am I crying, is it the ice inside melting?

This could be a cave, so deep, so dark. The cold is making me tired, I feel blurry I am lost.

FROM THE INSIDE OUT

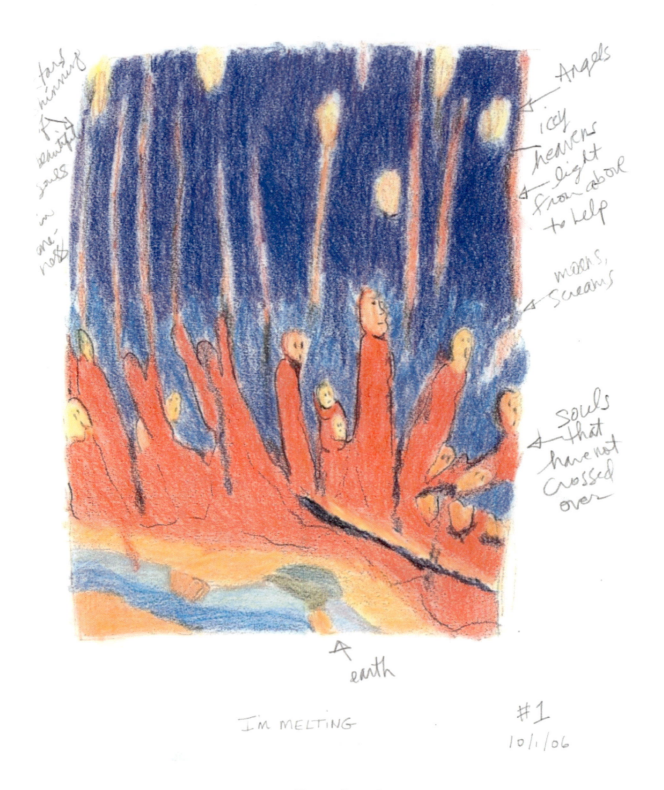

Drawing 1

Drawing Explanation: Painting 1 I'm Melting

At this time, two years after the accident, I didn't know where I ended physically or consciously. I felt constant pain and chaos on a cellular level and was aware of layers of existence much more vast then the mental mind could constantly and comfortably exist in. My mind was dwarfed by awareness of the confusion in the teeming life inside and expansive consciousness beyond it. Waves of pain spiraled out of control and a message of cellular wrongness and mental incapacity hummed in the background. The peace I knew from the near-death experience (NDE) was drowned out by scenes of fear, pain and loss.

Where did reality exist? My vision was turned inside and linked with a larger existence. The small "me" was fighting to right itself, creating fear while somewhere deep inside I knew peace. With continual pain, a separation was created where I could exist. I remember wanting peace more than anything else. The bombardment of information created chaos. I was drowning in it and existed in extreme overwhelm on all levels with one small quiet lifeline, the NDE. I couldn't contain myself. Parts of me were all over, scattering about. I was living dissolution and part of me was running in fear. I remember trying to move because moving meant aliveness. I had to be present and work at pulling myself together.

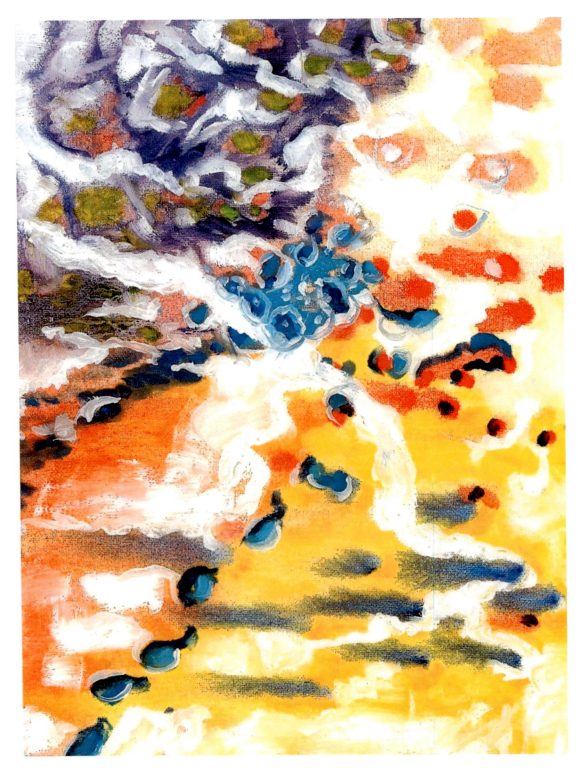

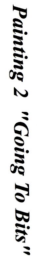
Painting 2 "Going To Bits"

Prose Painting 2   Going to Bits

I am inside an eggshell – I hear crunching.
I see bright lights that are too bright. I cannot see, I hear too loudly.

What is moving, what is still?

Bubbles are flying out of my head that belong inside.
I am losing the juice of life. It seeps out and things go crazy.
Sometimes things work and stop.
I don't know what is real.
I feel too much for this world but where am I?
Where do I go?
How do I move myself and stop?
Everything vibrates so when I move I have to get all of the layers to move, as if they trail behind me like a blurry photo. When I stop they keep on going and move through me, then shake back like jello.

I see this way, all shaky while I try to collect the scattering pieces.

All of the bits, going to bits and I don't want to be with other people or I will loose my bits and maybe take on theirs too.

Everything is such an effort.

I hear too much, it is painful.

Just being means feeling around for how to see, how to move how to find thinking.

Nothing feels good; nothing feels right, lost in nothingness unable to find my way out.

FROM THE INSIDE OUT

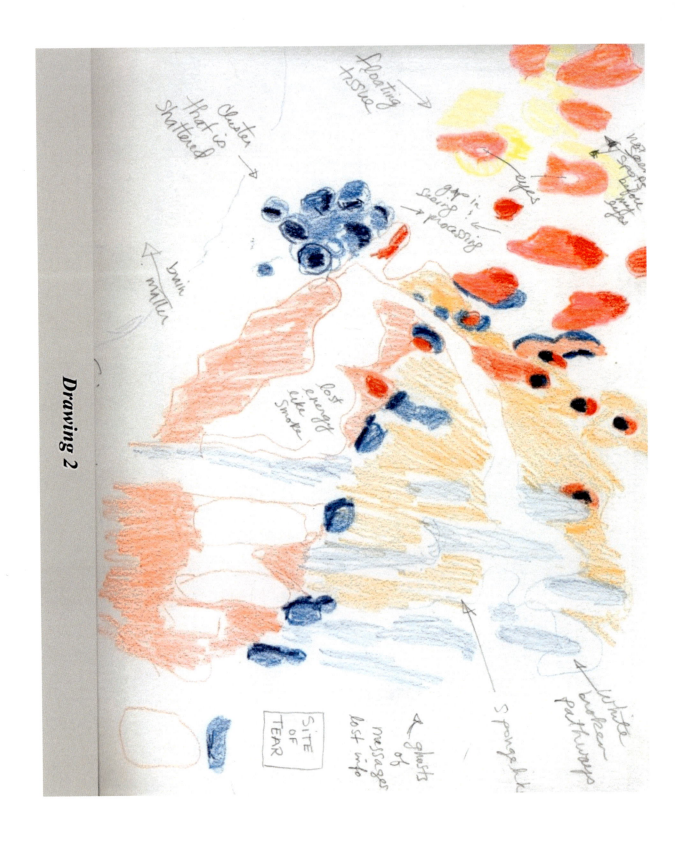

Drawing 2

Drawing Explanation: Painting 2 Going to Bits

During this time I felt as though I didn't and couldn't belong in this world. But I was also unsure where to go. My senses were magnified and life was incredibly painful. I felt there were no choices. It was impossible to stop the constant fear messages and chatter.

At University Hospital my occupational therapist, said the brain needed to be challenged or it would continue to shut down as much as possible. The challenges of numbers, reading and other worksheets she provided me with were painful and frustrating to attempt. I often had a numbing fear when I thought of walking the short distance to the little grocery store or library near my apartment. Dr. Landes, the psychologist on my team, coached me to learn how to examine the fear. Ask if it is life-threatening or something that would harm me. If it wasn't, then I could view it as the ego protecting itself and override the fear. I was very concerned that numbness and being frozen would happen at the worst times.

When visiting my dear friend in Pittsburgh I was pushing my brain by painting. We took a drive to an overlook of the hills of Pittsburgh and rode a cable car down a steep hill. I had an anxiety attack that day. I learned that looking from atop hills and airplane windows was to be avoided. My brain couldn't sort the information.

On some level I was acutely aware of my cells and I heard them. This awareness switched my brain back and forth from my cells to the greater universe. My personal map wasn't that of a compact body but rather of floating cells that wandered and external forces that entered my general body area. I tried to keep track of my cells because I was afraid they would drift off. The intensity of this information put me into sensory overload.

I still can't begin to imagine how I could paint this occurrence. It was overly abundant with rich sensory information that constantly changed.

The trauma to my brain impacted me visually. The neuro-ophthalmologist I saw, said that both of my eyes were moving side to side and forward and backward constantly like a camera lens. The doctor's information was a revelation to me. I finally understood the constant stress I felt when my eyes were open.

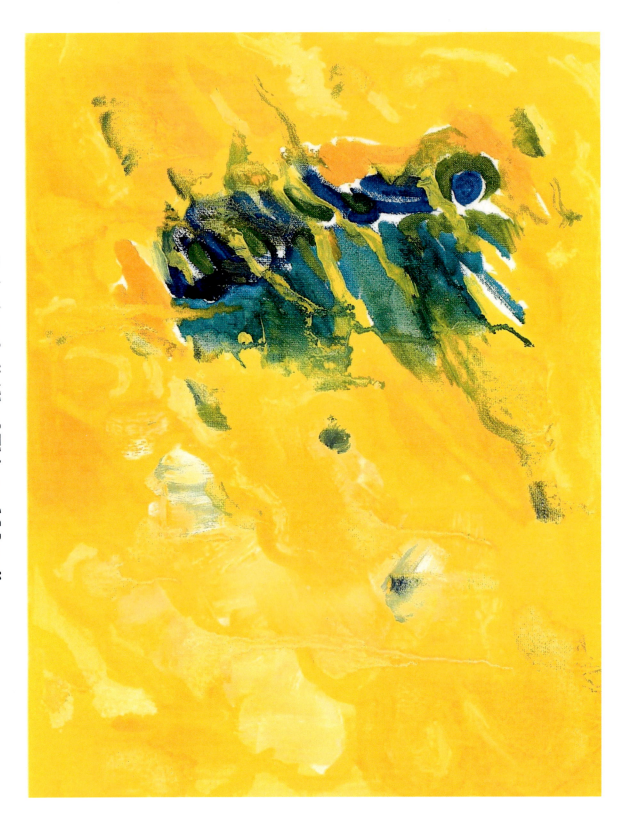

Painting 3 "All of This and More"

Prose Painting 3   All of This and More

Some things hang together.

Maybe those things are me.

Ice and bright cold lights they jar me. Wherever I move it follows. Eyes watching me from everywhere. Deep inside the Knower remembers but how to find the Knower.

Just a pile of bones and fish scales blowing in the wind, cooked under the hot sun.

How do you freeze from the heat?
Parts of me dance away - do they come back?
When I put something in my pocket it falls through like cents (sense?) lost falling out.

My eyes see everything yet I go nowhere. All of this and more.

FROM THE INSIDE OUT

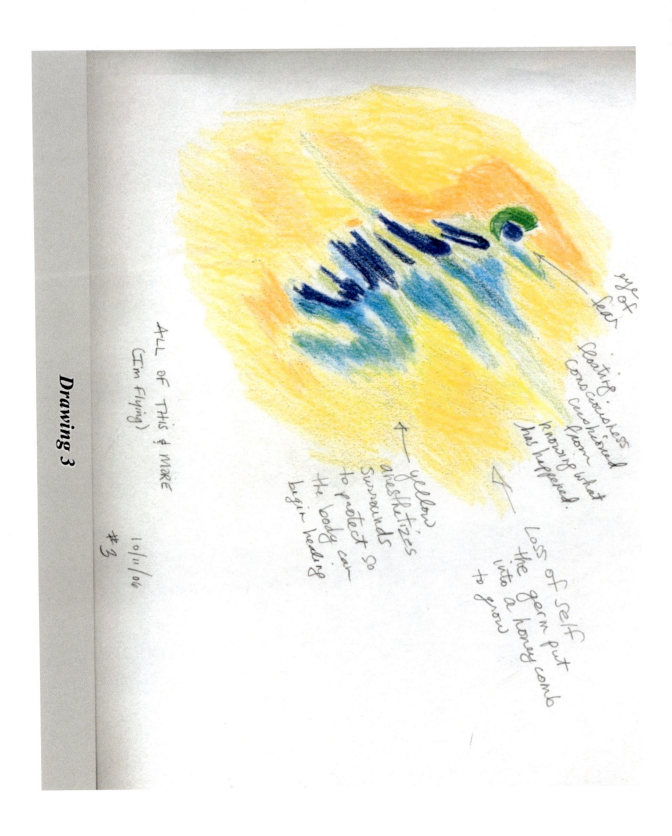

Drawing 3

Drawing Explanation: Painting 3 All of This and More

This was a time of acute contradictions. With the overwhelming sensitivities I was unable to process data. The middle ground was lost along with the ability to sift through information and do something with it. The way through the maze was just out of reach. I sensed it nearby yet millions of miles away. I knew that my awareness was running rampant, collecting tons of unusable information. Unusable because the filing systems were out of order. This time period felt like a catch-22. I existed; therefore part of the operating system was working, but compensating for a downed system by working overtime. Somehow the timer got stuck when the accident happened. I had a sense that I should have known the accident was about to happen and that I could have done something about it. The hidden assumption was that I didn't use more of my awareness to collect data that would have stopped or moderated the accident. Because my systems felt so compromised and vulnerable, data collection was working overtime to provide data and prevent another accident. My sense of safety and security in myself had evaporated.

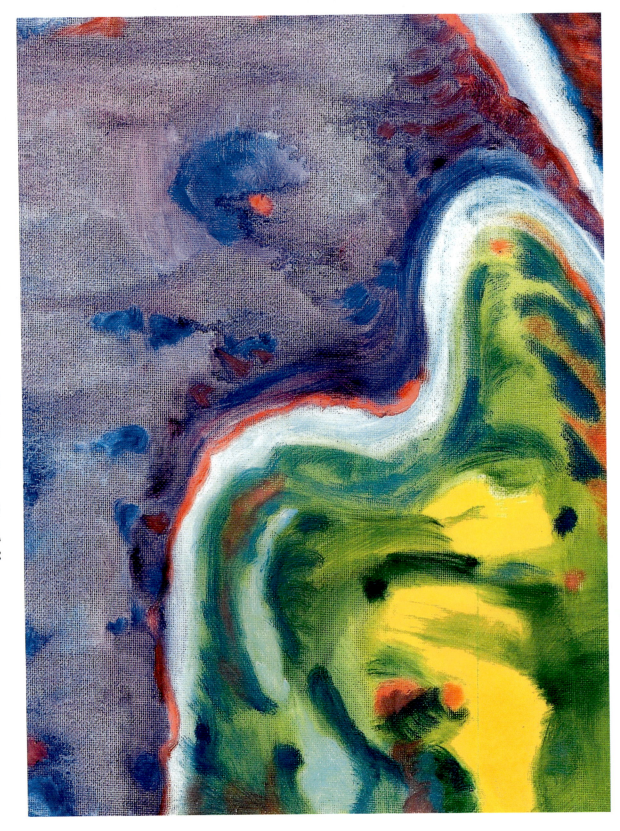

Painting 4 "A Broken Path"

Prose Painting 4   A Broken Path

Movement stops, sputters, searches for places to enliven. Scattered signals, missed flashes. Darkness, starkness, too bright and too dark all at once.

I feel growth sprouting, searching.

Is this what it is like to be born – to grow or sprout? Like tree rings, circles of age, of being dashed away.

Time has no meaning nor do I.

Embracing the pain, it is close, it is something and I know not what lies beyond shrouded in pulses of dullness.

A thick groggy curtain with holes. Does it protect me or hurt me? Are all of the impulses closed in to emanate out unleashed?

I follow the road and sometimes things stop and I think it is nowhere and it is bliss.

There is something I am supposed to know but I do not know how to find it, or to feel behind the pain and fog.

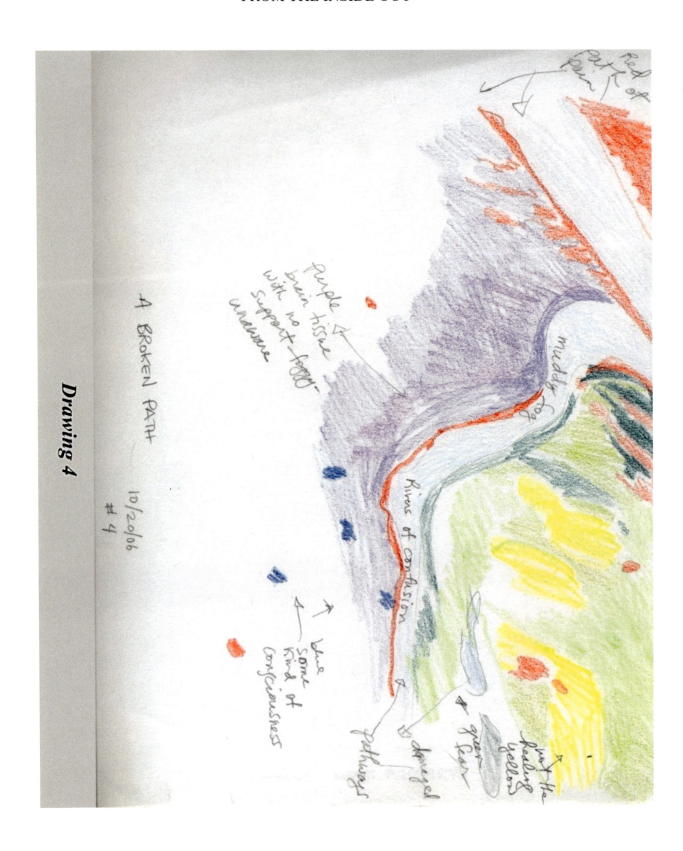

Drawing 4 — A BROKEN PATH 10/20/06 #4

CARA MAYO

Drawing Explanation: Painting 4 A Broken Path

This painting represents a duality to me: the deep-blue splotches of consciousness in contrast to the rivers of confusion and unaware foggy areas. There were times when I was very aware of the razor edge between each extreme.

My desire was to increase consciousness and the hope that was blooming and to stay out of pain and confusion so they wouldn't wash away healing. That desire in itself could set up a dynamic of stress. How interesting that life became a direction, not a goal, of driving my vehicle in the least stressful way while pushing for growth. Trial and error.

Again Dr. Landes eased my stress by telling me that if I pushed my brain too hard it wouldn't break but I would have symptoms to deal with. And I needed to push in order to work my way out. Balance became my key focus and I lived in a give-and-take way. Push and stretch, release and relax, heal, pat myself on the back, hug my struggling cells, look for other support, don't listen to any negativity, especially my own. I had to leave or not enter chaotic situations, and there were landmines of them in daily life from the chaos of TV and fluorescent lights to the murky thoughts around others. I went back to nature for a clear space.

Simplicity and gratitude rated high alongside balance. I added a large dose of creativity to find ways to achieve something rather than asking others for help. This direction represented the biggest gain. I accomplished something through my own independent action at my own rate and released myself from dealing with assumptions and expectations from myself and others.

My goal was independence using positive means that I could create or discover. I just knew there would be hard work involved, lots of little steps, but I knew the best solution was within reach. And so it continues to go. The brain is a muscle of awareness in the flow of life.

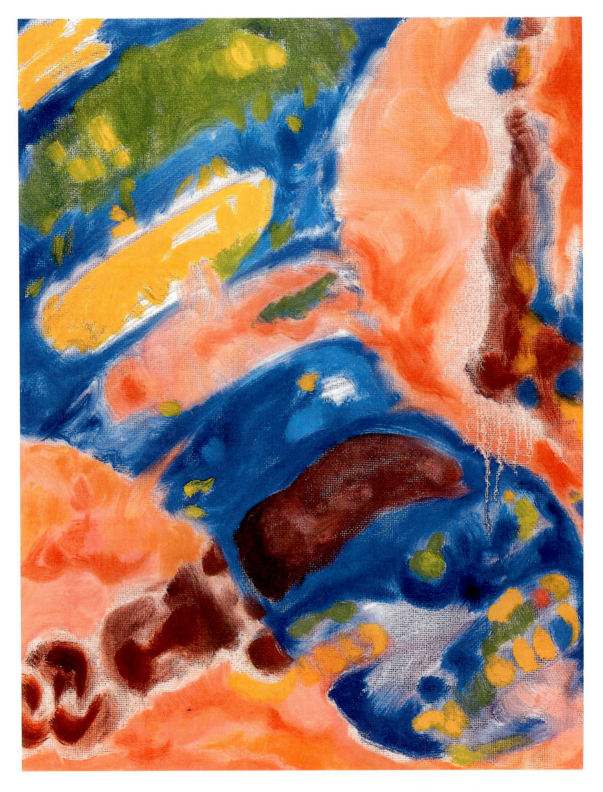

Painting 5 "Somewhere Beats a Heart"

Prose Painting 5   Somewhere Beats a Heart

Glows and deadness surround me.
I am caught in a broken vessel.
Smoke and steam cause friction hiding passage.
How to move and bond with another part that functions.
How to fire systems up that threaten to short circuit with overload.

Some places overwhelm me to remind me of life. It is like being nudged by a nagging child.

I long for sleep, deep sleep, to drift away gently.

There is nothing gentle here.

Everything screams or feels dead or lost. The pulsing must follow some pattern that is bigger than this organism called me. I bow in recognition to those things greater than knowing.

Like a pearl hidden in the depths of a rigid frame I slowly wiggle to find what supports me.

Yes, I am deep down under this growing slowly so that I can come out.

I hope that I can come out and be protected.
My skin is too new, two pink.
My eyes are blind with darkness or light. Maybe someone can see my bubbles.

FROM THE INSIDE OUT

Drawing 5

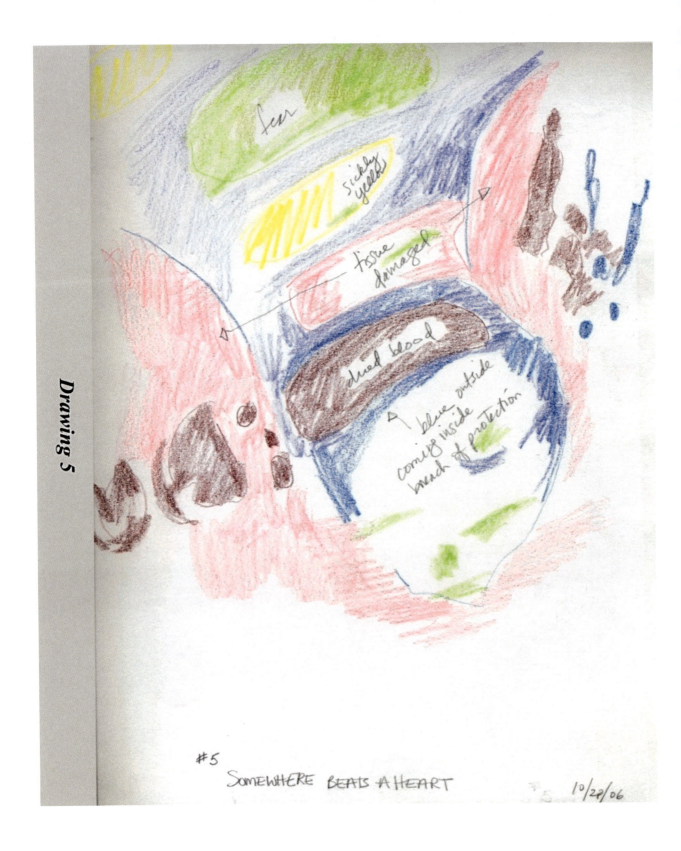

#5 SOMEWHERE BEATS A HEART 10/28/06

Drawing Explanation: Painting 5 Somewhere Beats a Heart

I remember feeling, "I am alive deep down inside here and I hope someone sees it so that people don't give up on me." I really needed a reflection of recognition for the conscious part of me that was totally overwhelmed by pain and survival. I didn't like what I saw and I worried about what others saw.

Eight months after the accident I went to University Hospital in Syracuse, N.Y. The staff and doctors who I saw were a primary support system for me, as was my friend Rosanne and cousin Eileen. They accepted that I was doing the best I could. They expected me to recover in my own time and they cared for me with no expectations or assumptions. To me it was unconditional love. Their reflection helped me ease up on myself and put energy into releasing stress and healing. It was extremely important to spend some time around them. The saving grace was my support systems.

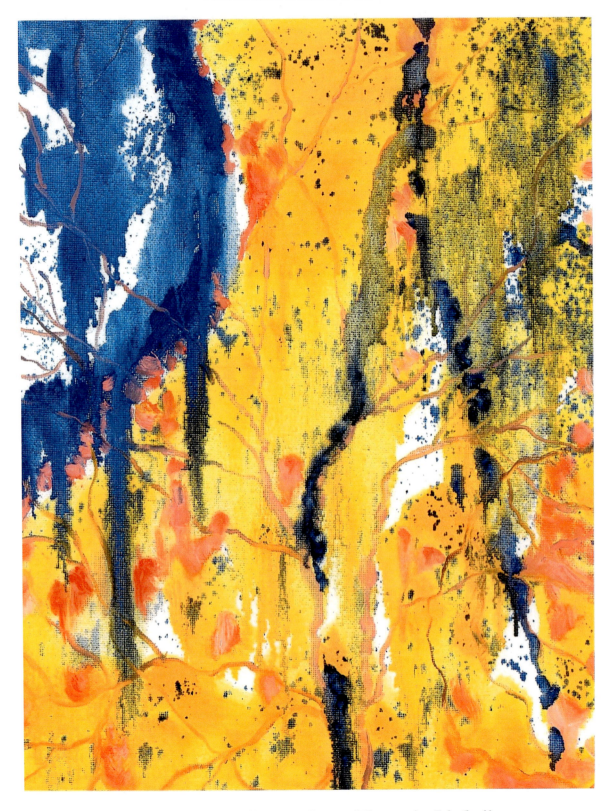

Painting 6 "Somewhere There is Light"

Prose Painting 6 Somewhere There is Light

Red drips muted, sinking into sponge.

Sinkholes and crevasses where there were none.

Holes for insects to hide in.

A time when new signals reach out.
Their searching is the breath of life.
I breathe knowing something has connected.

There is a broken mirror and I use it to signal for help.

Is anyone there?

Put away the map, start over. Wander and hold on to every flash of life.

Somewhere there is Light.

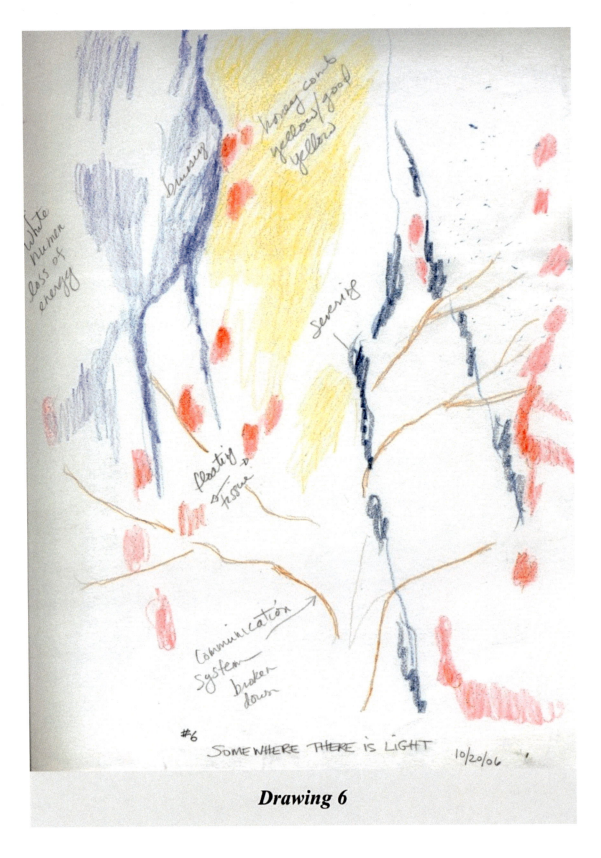

Drawing 6

Drawing Explanation: Painting 6 Somewhere There Is Light

The insects hiding represented my fear about hidden damage physically, emotionally, mentally and spiritually. I still wonder about this today and return to the simplicity of nature to release stress and feel gratitude to move through these fears when they flare up. Total memory loss of a situation and other issues that arise now can bring fears to the surface. I try to use tools or get help to air out my subconscious. The concussion has made me more aware of the need to be responsible for any chaos or negativity I have and to rout it out, reformat to a positive message and stay vigilant.

I felt like the little Dutch boy that plugged up the dam with his fingers. I knew that I had a mine zone of sponge holes, crevasses and sinkholes that threatened my vehicle constantly. The desire for some security, some terra firma, kept me moving. I did know that there were constant pitfalls in my previous life or future healed life. I just wanted to create an island to stand on where I could breathe and work from. In the meantime I was constantly searching for support, whether it was the song of a bird outside my window or a smile from a stranger. I did believe in the constant spiral toward wholeness out of chaos. I counted on the extra push toward wholeness and leaned back into it for support. It didn't matter where this idea came from. I could protect my back, feel universal support and have a thrust block to push off from. Another golden star to support healing.

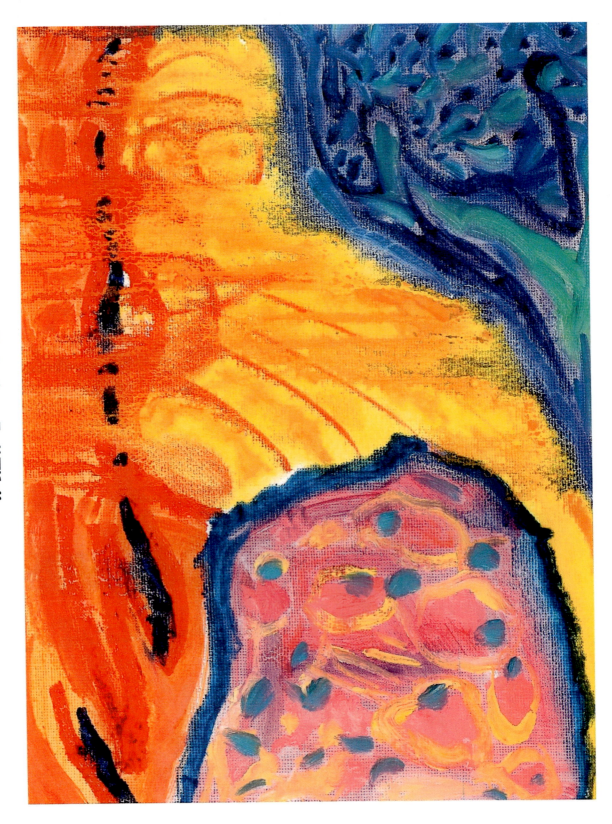

Painting 7 "Tilt"

Prose Painting 7   Tilt

One area can look different, chopped up, compartmentalized. Many things going on at once, competing for attention.

Confusion..........confusion.........the next step is tilt or shut down.

How to subdue all of the info and find what I need to attend to.

Chaos threatening to engulf me.

I so dislike the noise of chaos and long for peace and contentment. The constant struggle against chaos can create more. Desire is to bundle extraneous info and caste it away. Must retrain brain to filter.

Fear of being carried away into insanity which is loss of self.

Noise of chaos drowns out clear, small voices of connection to the Universe - Beingness.

FROM THE INSIDE OUT

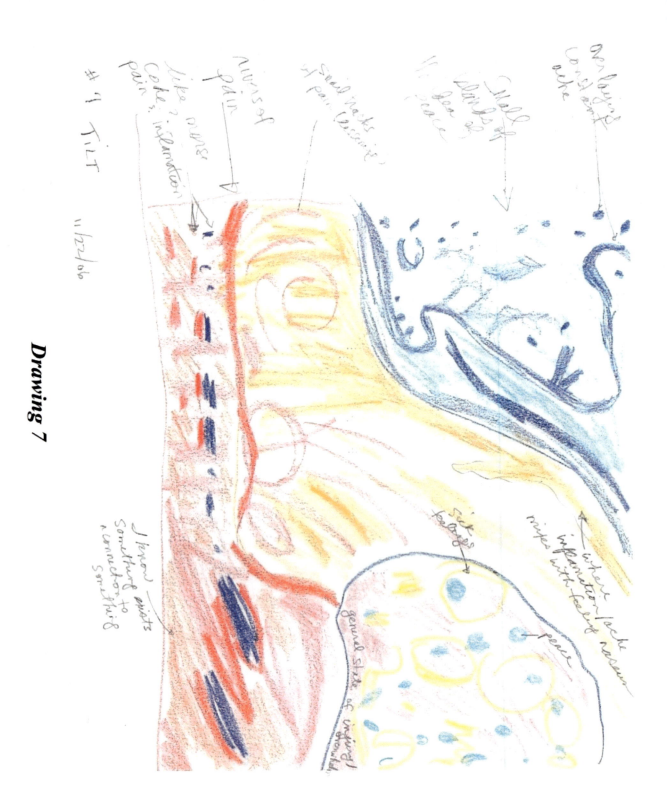

Drawing 7

Drawing Explanation: Painting 7 Tilt

In this painting I was concerned with the noise of chaos. Thoughts arose of locusts filling the sky and landing on a field where the crunching was loud and audible. Then the locusts would fly off, leaving barren desolation behind. I was afraid of what would be left behind. Whether my brain remained fuzzy or I had more clarity of desolation, either thought was frightening.

I knew peace existed. At this time a very small, quiet voice inside was shouting over the crunching. Like parting rows of beaded curtains I searched behind for small pads of peace. I want to think we all have peace hardwired into us, and sometimes it takes patience to find it.

I also want to think that every precious moment I stopped mental chatter helped the pools of peace deepen and grow. I learned over and over that increasing peace meant focusing on what I wanted. That is why I strongly believe that concussions create brain chaos and the best way to reduce brain stress and encourage healing is to focus on simple positive emotions.

I started with a brief reminder of something positive—the deeper the positive emotion the better. Then the slow, regular act of quieting the mind, if possible, followed. Listening to nature helps. His Holiness the Dalai Lama, Mother Theresa and Gandhi suggested that we focus on peace, not on eradicating war.

The simple steps are meditative practices that have been around for a long time. Sitting with people that are meditating helps. Just the vibration of calmness can help quiet a concussive person. This happened when I was with my friend Rosanne. She has hospice experience, was a head nurse and trained in alternative therapy.

I always received love, comfort, peace and the reflection that I was okay from Rosanne. I really needed that constant support, not in words so much but in being-ness. Insanity represented the fever pitch of chaos. I knew from the NDE that complete dissolution of consciousness doesn't happen until we enter the Void.

With the ego running rampant I expended a lot of energy to move through and overcome the egoic voices. It felt like my body was deeply in shock and overbalanced wildly on the survival side. I eventually had conversations with my cells, quieting them and telling them we were healing. I think the visual problems I had were traceable to the desire to see everything all at once and protect myself.

Again the answer nestled in strengthening my intuition. With hypersensitive senses and ego gone wild the only real protection I had was my intuition. The way to intuition was through peace and clearing a place to hear or sense intuition. I still perceived myself as always moving, a blurred, shaking, loose conglomerate of frantic cells. The feeling of moving into the flow was where I found intuition. Therefore I would move slower than the frantic wobbling but I moved with something that I perceived as greater than myself.

The moments I moved into this larger flow added layers of such being-ness that felt like perfection to me. Trying to stop the chaos created more chaos. Moving into the present moment with deliberateness and intention created spaces of healing. I wasn't fighting, I was moving from the inside out, gradually slowing the movement down, trying to turn the tide. I only hoped I was close to reaching critical mass. Knowing what lay behind me (layers of chaos) pushed me to continue.

I was afraid that if I stopped and hunkered down, the chaos and fear would eclipse and engulf me. Perhaps for others hunkering down into a den would be more helpful. For my personality it wasn't. Active participation moving into intuition or flow helped me become stronger. The lesson of security by moving with the flow is my desired way of life now. It doesn't mean constant physical movement, rather shifting through the balance of physical, mental, emotional and spiritual growth.

The message I have is of constant change, in some way. Security, while changing, is provided through my intuition, which also flows. Suddenly I'm not existing in a hardened structure. This mutually consenting conglomerate of cells, with the added dash from mental, emotional and spiritual states, all connect to the universe.

Now when I do something I watch myself doing it rather than living in a predominantly mental way. There is a synergy and my intuition can override everything. Because I know I can't possibly be consciously aware of all of the facets of a situation, intuition sorts through to bring things together and I use other tools for completion.

The concussion forced me to simplify and live deeper.

CARA MAYO

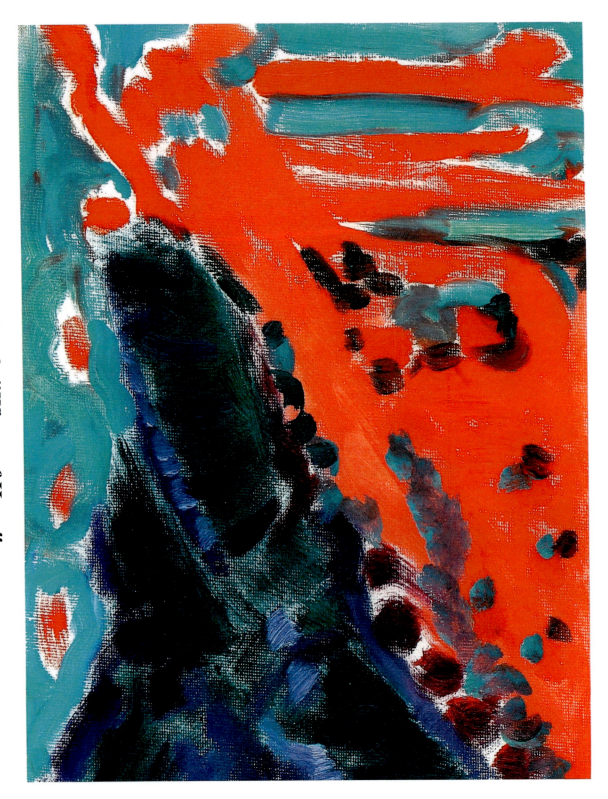

Painting 8 "Wings of Hope"

Prose Painting 8   Wings of Hope

Flood of pain threatens to erode peace/contentment.

Wings of struggle work hard to hold up the place of prayer/meditation.
Unable to meditate, can't find it, how to do it?

Only to stop incredible slide of pain, fear, chaos that equals nothingness, loss of self. And would a 'whole' return or be something else or someone else?

Wings -refusal to let go of self-hood. Struggle to hold and eventually emerge. Focus on knowingness of return of self-hood.

Realization of fear re-creates and works toward chaos.

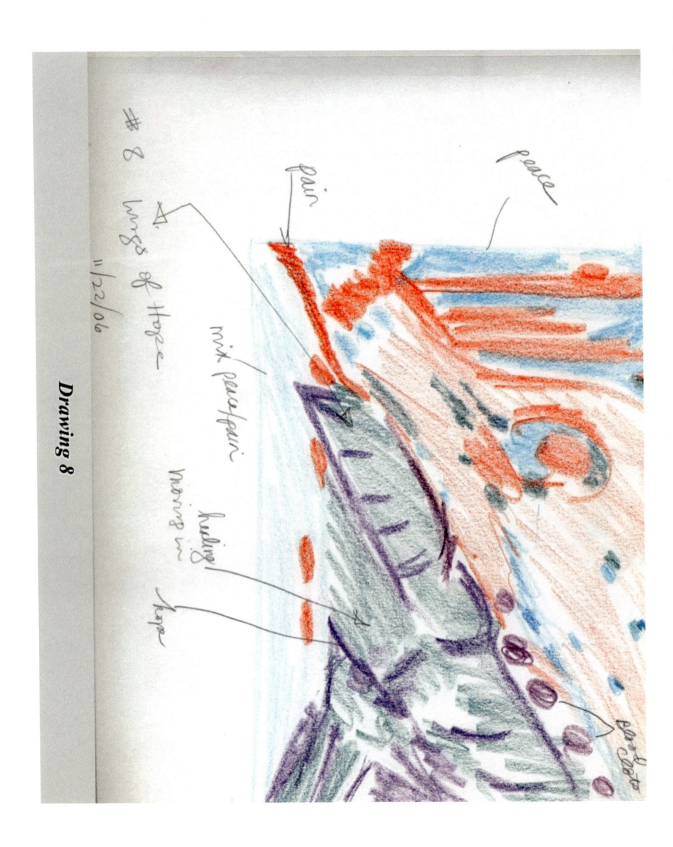

Drawing 8

Drawing Explanation: Painting 8 Wings of Hope

In this painting the areas of peace are getting stronger and growing. While I was concerned about the tide turning, it already had. Fuzziness was evaporating and the stark contrast between peace and pain served as a clear reminder. Like the grooved pavement along the shoulder of a road I now had instant feedback. At the time the contrast was overwhelming and I didn't perceive the degree of healing it represented. When the murky gloom lifted it was a slow, steady recession and it is still occurring today.

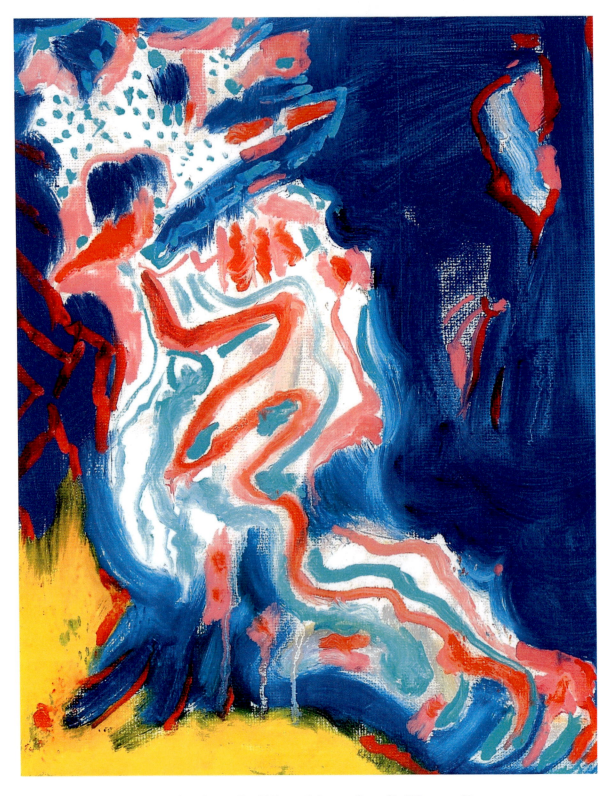

Painting 9 "Looking for Stillness"

Prose Painting 9   Looking for Stillness

Contrasts of pain and peace.

A sick feeling numbed by darkness.

What is the best? The sick feeling because I know I exist or the numbing darkness?

Is it possible to hold onto the pain and peace together to create a stillness?

Is there a space in time I can cocoon to heal?

More is happening now. There is movement. It takes all of my strength and more to do this.

I know something is helping me.

Is it my cells trying to re-connect to the Universe, to Oneness? Their quiet workings are like a white river of mist.

I hope it is there – I need it to be there. Just out of reach is another level of information. Something I am not used to but it exists.

How to find it, be conscious of it.............

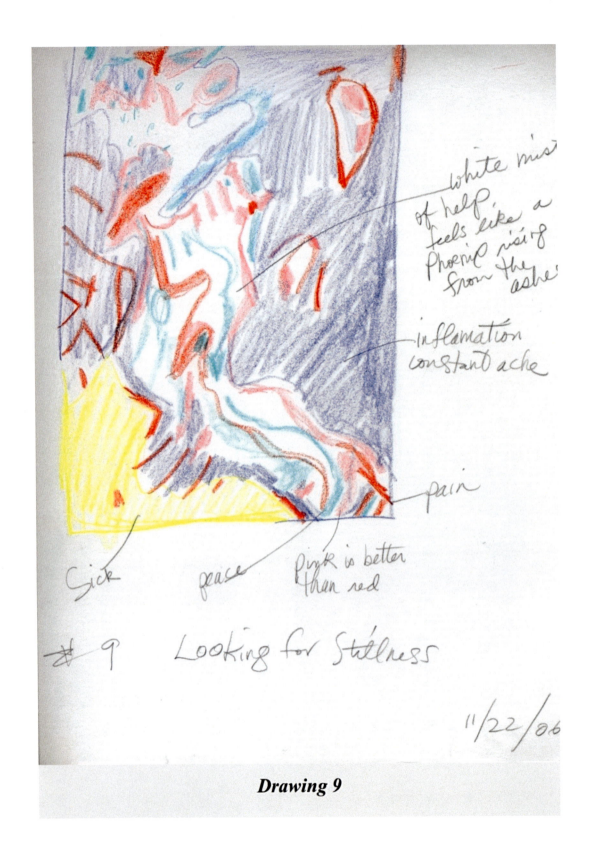

Drawing 9

Drawing Explanation: Painting 9 Looking For Stillness

Here the movement is stronger. Something is very obviously happening. I know there is a positive thrust for healing but still I am tested severely. On this level, movement and change have lifted me from my usual pattern. I am unsure of where to be, what is happening, how to help and what to hold onto. The feeling of being stretched, the "no pain, no gain" idea, is squarely facing me. I felt frozen with the need to be ever ready, to stay vigilant and alert yet not sink into stress or rest in the pain. Even the thought of holding on to the coattails of velvety pink Pepto-Bismol pain called to me. At least I could rest in it and know I was somewhere. My visual of stretching everything out to find the next handhold waiting for me, putting my ultimate fate and knowing on the line, existed for me here. It felt forever, a lifetime, and I asked for help.

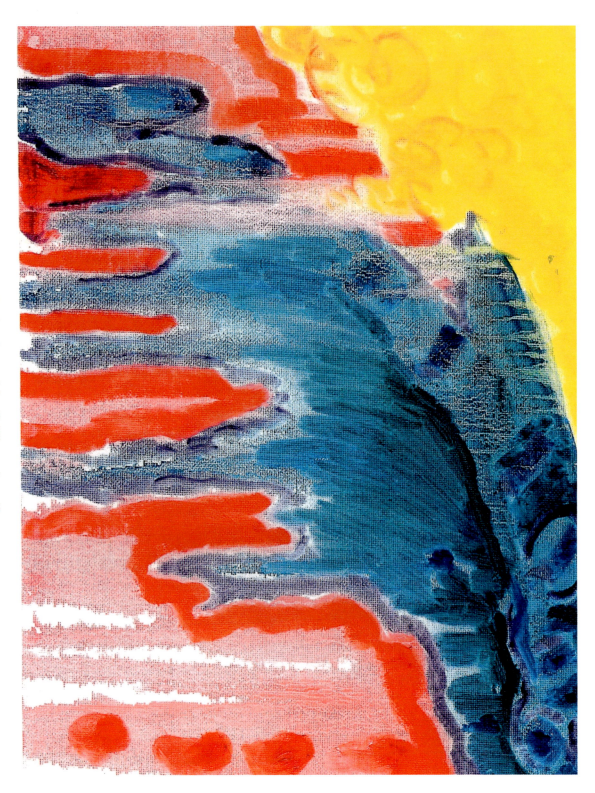

Painting 10 "Clearing"

Prose Painting 10   Clearing

The swirls of yellow are like billowing smoke. The wind is blowing it away....... Feather of healing pushing the air.

Vibrations from this feather go down into the injured parts.

I feel movement, like the wings of a hummingbird.
Quiet, small but changing things some how. I just know there is change.
It feels big, I want it to be big, to keep going.

For now I reach inside to sense the change, to be a Watcher.

I see myself open up and breathe deeply to let more change fill me.

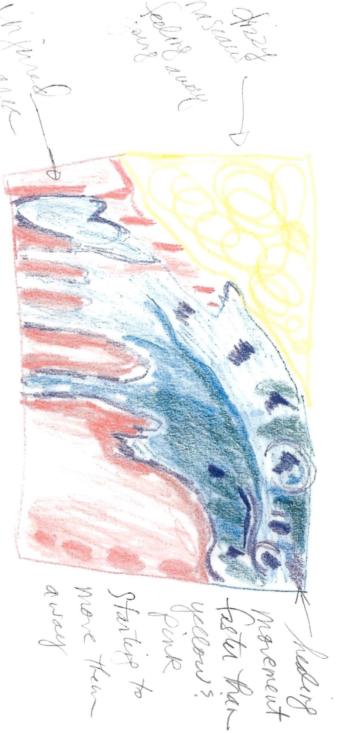

Drawing 10

Drawing Explanation: Painting 10 Clearing

At this point I am aware of the movement of healing that is happening and I can embrace the feeling. I spent time searching inside to find, or since the positive changes even to feel, the cell as it shifts from chaos. I was awestruck by the sheer number of minute movements. Like a constant breeze evaporating water, the healing wind ceaselessly fanned out the feelings of chaos. I was still working from the other side, reassuring my body that I was safe creating as calm and stress-free an environment as possible.

Holding, cradling an injured area, talking to it reassuringly and listening for a response of how I could ease pain and increase healing came into play here. Having set the stage, the door was open for messages to come through my intuition and send me toward another step along the path of healing. I did have some very intuitive information that helped with the balance of reducing stress and challenges.

There was nothing easy about this process. In May 2005 my older son was in Florence, Italy. It seemed to be the only time for me to pursue a lifelong dream of traveling to Italy. Dr. Landes asked me if I thought it was a good thing to do. I had to go. My brother traveled with me. Flying was horribly painful but I had a technique to use, learned from a class taken the weekend before departure. I asked for internal help continually throughout the trip.

Every moment of the trip was a challenge and there was no way and nowhere to give up. Somehow I took pictures and constantly talked to myself to work with dizziness and nausea. Looking through a camera at the leaning Tower of Pisa almost left me lying in the grass. Unfortunately my constant companions of dizziness and nausea and eye issues cut back on my enjoyment of the wonderful food, shopping, art museums and other things that all needed what I was lacking: the ability to focus.

I kept moving and absorbing just like I had for the 11 months prior. So much energy was spent monitoring all systems that a part of me normally covered in layers was free to dance with life. Even though I didn't grasp names, directions, language and much of what was going on around me, I was experiencing the feeling of the places I visited. And while my son was in charge of arrangements, I felt secure to go places on my own. Intuition was directing me.

An interesting realization occurred when I was having a conversation with my son. Jared speaks some Italian, and my brother and I have a vestige of Spanish from high school. There were two Italian men in their late 20s sitting across from us on a bus. As usual I was doing a simple vibrational technique to keep symptoms in check, feeling consumed by this necessity. Later that day I asked my son what the two men said, knowing they made some remarks while watching him talk to two American women.

FROM THE INSIDE OUT

While on the bus I gave the two men the eye, staring at them to make them uncomfortable. Jared concurred with my feeling about the remarks from the men and said he was keeping an eye on them also. There I was seemingly in my own world but understanding what was unfolding. It happened throughout the trip. I was totally present, coping instant to instant. No one noticed that I always touched walls beside me or kept my hand on something stable. They didn't notice the times I closed my eyes behind sunglasses under a big hat to calm symptoms, perhaps thinking I was resting.

The trip represented a huge challenge but I learned so much from it. When I returned home I decided to find out how long I could keep my eyes open without pain. It came to three hours a day. After three hours, brain stress increased and not in a linear fashion. We wandered around Italy for three weeks, and I not only survived but filled myself with incredible beauty.

CARA MAYO

FROM THE INSIDE OUT

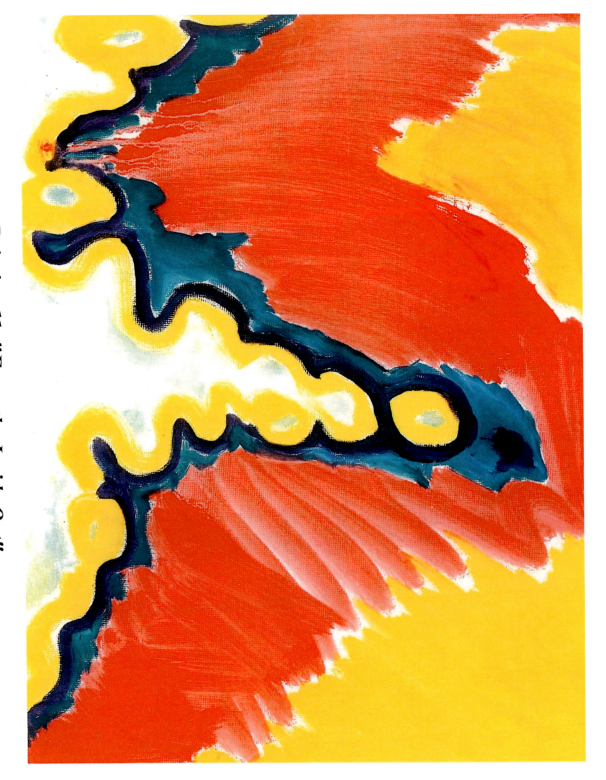

Painting 11 "From the Inside Out"

Prose Painting 11   From the Inside Out

Bubbles of frosting, white movement of healing move up from inside.

Blue flames of healing burn away the sickness.

Angry area, still injured are a contrast to the vibrant movement that arrests and eclipses the injured parts.

The germ of healing (purple spot) heads the movement. It pushes and expands moving faster than the slow stagnant injured area.

Like a flame racing through me, soon I will breathe more deeply.

Soon I will reclaim more of who I am that was hidden by pain.

And I wonder what will be there after the purging flame clears out the heavy suffocating blankets.

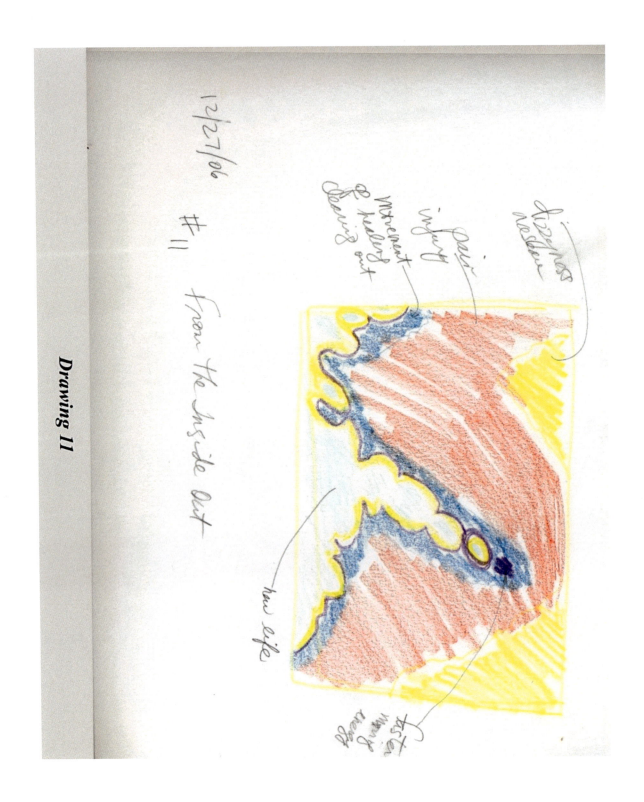

Drawing 11

Drawing Explanation: Painting 11 From the Inside Out

One of my earliest thoughts focused on the superpowers I would emerge with after healing was completed. I remember telling Dr. Landes that I was still looking for my superpowers. They were right with me the entire way.

The superpower of the natural direction toward progress as a contrast to chaos was there. We all have this. The superpower of other areas taking up extra duties to compensate for injuries. And we have internal suggestions toward living a better life. It may mean digging really deep or watching what arises in the simplest way. There is preciousness for very small things that I didn't bother with before.

And the "world in a mustard seed" realization was prominent during healing. I can value a small thing in nature and feel I have the riches of the world. Maybe it is most important to release what is thought to be valuable. Start from scratch.

It was wonderfully valuable to me to be able to go for a walk. I experienced the riches around me. Did the passing jogger feel that way? Who knows? I was on my path and I was grateful for what I had.

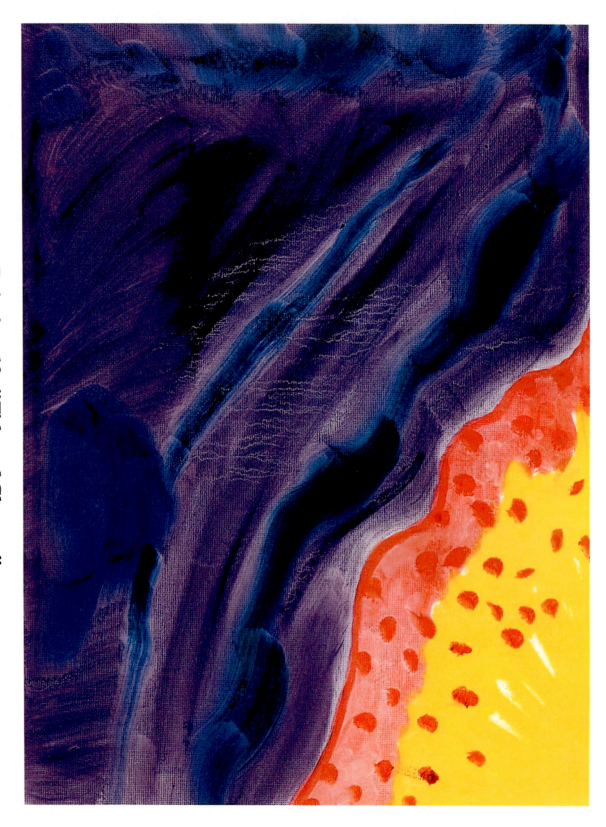

Painting 12 "Tides of Change"

Prose Painting 12   Tides of Change

Like water ever moving the healing pushes over areas of injury cleansing and healing them.

It is a strong force bathing the area in pure, strong light and vibration.

Like an army marching, the tide has turned. Different waves of healing move in.

Some for calming to ease the chaos, others for cleansing and the deep purple for higher vibration and faster movement.

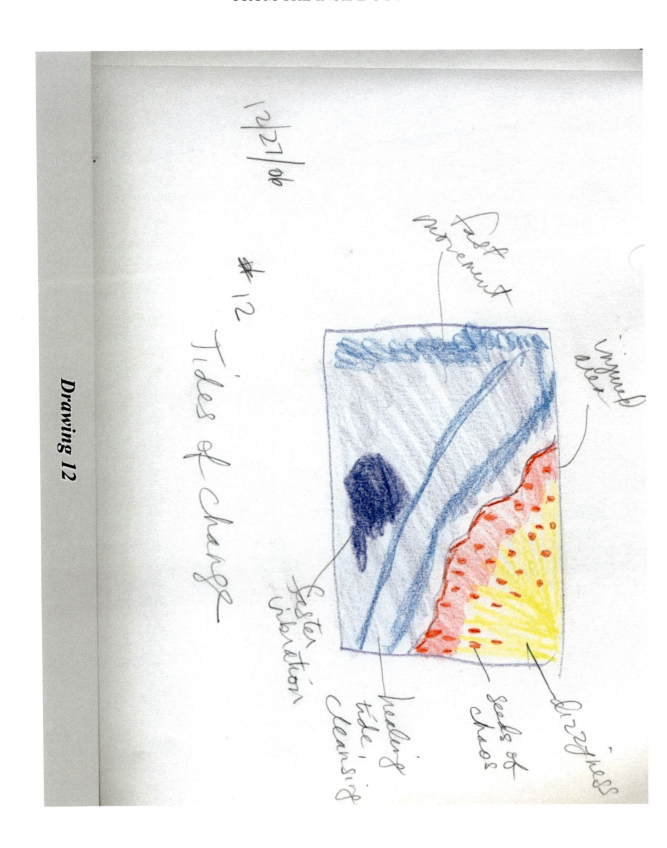

Drawing 12

Drawing Explanation: Painting 12 Tides of change

At this time I know the cleansing moving through me has taken over. While vestiges of damage remain, the power of change is unknowable. And so I watch to see how I will emerge. I wonder what the new "me" is. How do I find what is here and what is gone? And I know that after the purple tide is gone a new world awaits me. I dream, I hope to learn and emerge as more than who I was, more authentic. And I wonder how I can access the unknown or unused parts of my brain. That too is my direction; having come from emptiness all things are possible.

"Having come from emptiness all things are possible." That is how I intend to continue living my life. Healing from the concussion hasn't stopped. I realize that now that less energy is directly focused on concussion symptoms and more on body and systems balance. What I accepted as health prior to August 2004 is no longer acceptable. I settled for the norm and aimed a little above it. There is so much more movement, healing, balance and synergy available. I want to continue experiencing and uncovering those superpowers. The new frontier is always me. I know the healthier I become, the more I give others. I would like to help myself and others as much as possible. It is not a lazy journey. To be ever vigilant, flow with change, rest in the support around me, be authentic and live bigger with the universe; that is my goal.

Chapter 2

During the middle years of my recovery from TBI (2007 to 2015) I moved five times in the Northern Virginia area. Driving in Northern Virginia was a constant challenge for me. Other than a few previous trips through the area, everything was new to me. It was a very dense, bustling, crowded area. I had moved to be near my sons but they were very busy working. Living 12 miles away from them was often enough of an impediment to seeing each other frequently. I walked a great deal and, because I was unable to manage the Metrorail system or buses, I spent most of my time alone.

On my daily walking route in Old Town Alexandria I came upon a Tibetan Buddhist meeting place. Drawn by the quiet, soothing energy I began attending. It was a haven with people pausing to meditate, to be present and to support each other. It was that rare place where people were nonjudgmental—each focused on their own journey. It was the only place I felt supported and not judged. While I wasn't able to quiet my mind and meditate, I could repeat a prayerful mantra and feel the peace and gratitude around me. The ritual and verses were beyond my ability to comprehend, but when I settled into the richness that filled my senses and heart I felt grateful. It was a respite from the constant fear.

At that time I began reciting mantras so that I could drive and maneuver through life. There were times of exhilaration when I felt in the flow of life. Reciting mantras helped me feel safer.

There were blissful days when I walked the 13 blocks into Old Town reciting mantras and telling myself I could have anything I wanted; clothes, shoes, a great meal, desert. I roamed the streets looking, watching and choosing to fill myself with prayer and gratitude for the abundance around me. It was a practice that shifted my awareness from lack to abundance.

Moving closer to my sons made it difficult to attend Tibetan Buddhist events in Alexandria. Mass transit was available but I had to take a Metrorail train and a bus, making it a very tiring day. I continued to attend until I moved farther away and the combination of driving farther in traffic and my flagging energy ended my attendance. I continue to recite mantras. A prayer or blessing is a better choice than brain noise.

Over the years personal management issues demanded most of my energy. I was in survival mode, fighting to maintain what I had and was losing. In the meantime, I also was unearthing more brain deficits. Hypervigilance and constant brain noise made life impossible to bear.

While my body attempted to heal, adrenal fatigue was a key factor in my downward slide. When I saw Dr. Landes in 2006, two years after the accident, I still had a vital body and I was very focused on pushing through and sorting out my injured brain. As the years passed my word and memory issues were slowly getting better while my body functioning showed the cumulative effects of adrenal fatigue.

Adrenal fatigue, as I learned in a 2015 blood draw, had continued over the years to stress my body functions. I was failing. In 2015 it took tremendous effort to go out two times a week. The rest of the time I was sitting on the couch tired and overwhelmed. My sleep was getting worse and everything took more effort. I saw myself fading into a future of having a significant illness and needing more care. I felt like I was out of options. As a last-ditch attempt I decided to move to a small, quiet area in the country.

Chapter 3

In 2015 I was at a point where I didn't know if I could continue. Life was getting harder to manage. My body was shutting down. It was time for a last-ditch attempt because I knew that not making a life change would lead to a significant illness.

I have never lived in a small town and longed for quiet. It was my hope that a smaller town would be less stressful and helpful in relieving the adrenal fatigue. My daughter-in-law suggested a small, artsy town near the Blue Ridge Mountains. A friend of mine, hearing about my dilemma with driving, offered to take me on an overnight trip to look at the area. When I saw the mountains I started to breathe, and driving home on Skyline Drive filled me with joy and a sense of freedom.

For a year I lived eight miles outside of a small town. The quiet and stars were wonderful. Driving into town each day proved to be taxing so I moved to an apartment close to the main area of town.

The first week after my initial move I volunteered to help refurbish an old building for the local art center. Volunteer work offset the feelings of fear I had living three hours from family and not knowing anyone in the community. I went through a time of feeling lost, abandoned and punished. I was very much alone and often went for drives in the countryside, becoming more comfortable getting lost and wandering.

The beauty around me, kind people, slower pace and low traffic density provided the stress reduction I needed.

It wasn't easy starting over. Better sleep and quiet time gave me a chance to objectively take stock. I wasn't happy with what I saw and it was apparent that I had to do something and create a life for myself with what I possessed at the time. Maybe I would continue to heal, maybe I wouldn't. How could I fashion a joyful life with what I had?

It wasn't as if my sensitivity to noise, fluorescent lights and memory issues went away. I still had to manage myself and face uncovering more problems but I could find quiet places to recharge.

Nature is a treasure and her richness feeds me. Along with the memories from my near-death experience, of being surrounded and filled with love, I have a foundation to support me.

The traumatic brain injury forced me to simplify my life. I remain aware of the energy around me and the choices I make. Slowly my resilience is increasing and I am steadily pushing outward at my own speed.

My biggest creation is reassembling myself, taking care of myself and having patience to do this as a devotional practice to Spirit.

Acknowledgements

Special thanks and gratitude to Jared Gruber, Oren Gruber, Joe Mayo, Rosanne Taylor and Ann McCartney—all part of my life before, during and after the accident—and to Cathy Minkler Gruber.

I was very fortunate to work with Dr. Allan Landes a year after the accident. His caring manner and wise words were a bedrock to me when I felt hopeless. He was instrumental in my healing and I found solace remembering what he told me.

Dr. Mark Gordon of Millennium Health Centers provided a basis for healing adrenal fatigue in 2015. I was at the end of my rope physically and didn't know where to turn.

I am deeply grateful to the many people who helped and supported me (and still do) through this recovery process from TBI. You know who you are.

My memory, while much better now, wasn't working for many years and still struggles. If I have overlooked anyone, please accept my heartfelt appreciation for the caring and support you provided me.

And lastly, I am very grateful to Wayne Drumheller, M.Ed., Editor and Founder of the Creative Short Book Writers Project, a collective of independently, published authors, experienced editors, teachers, educators, artisans, book mentors, and everyday people, who commit to professionally edit and publish books, and build a local and regional legacy in fiction and nonfiction literary excellence, and his "Writing As Art, Editing & Publishing" workshop at the Waynesboro Public Library that inspired and encouraged me to write, edit and publish this work.

About the Paintings

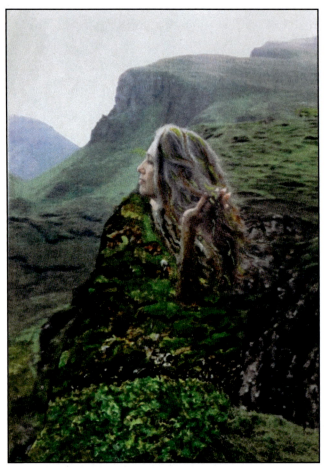

The paintings in this book emerged from a process honed for more than three decades. Art has always been my primary mode of expression. Art classes and clubs in junior high and high school led to a Bachelor of Fine Arts degree, work in technical illustration, mapmaking, jewelry repair, teaching art and continued art education over the years.

The process of artwork and writing was a natural expansion of making preparatory sketches and notes, a skill learned in middle school. About 14 years before the accident, I began a disciplined daily meditation practice and study that continued until the accident. Additionally my child and adult near-death experiences contributed to my continual, internal spiritual exploration. The combined focus of these long-standing practices pushed through the rubble of a nonfunctional brain and struggling physical body.

The desire to learn and explore overrode limitations and flowed in a time-honed process. Ignoring nausea, dizziness, eyestrain and headaches I painted during the darkness and quiet of night, turning inward to allow information to flow through me. The paintings, poems and drawings arose.

This compilation represents a time of suffering and expansion. It reveals to me the importance of focusing a long-term quest through disciplined practices. The slow emergence from chaos toward healing visible in Painting 9, showed me the moment my awareness re-engaged. It was a miracle caught on canvas.

The paintings on the following pages (My Gallery) display artwork created before the accident (2004), during the middle years of my healing (2005-2015) and current artwork (2016-2018). They are included to give the reader a broader perspective of my journey as an artist.

My Gallery: 2004, Before the Accident

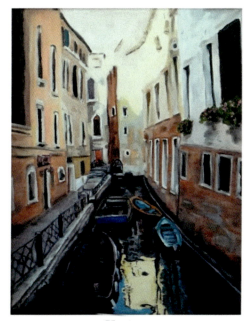
Venice

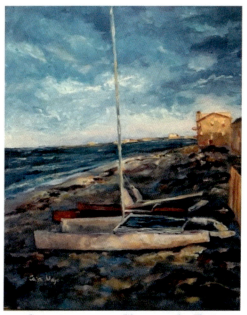
Catamarans on Chesapeake Bay

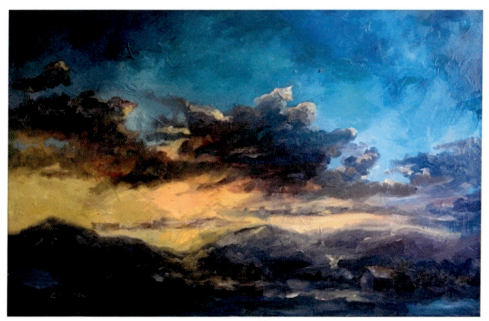
Mom's Sky

FROM THE INSIDE OUT

Paintings from: 2005 - 2015

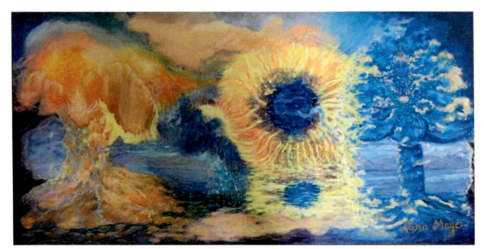

NDE Journey

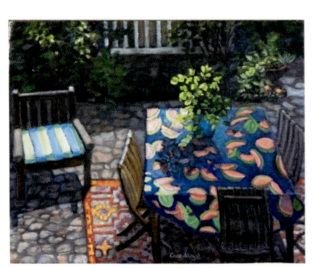

The Garden

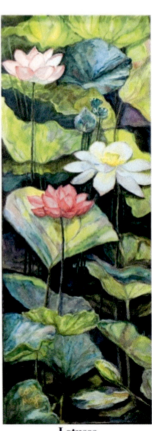

Lotuses

Artwork from: 2016 - 2018

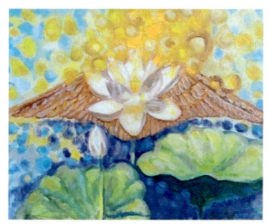

Golden Lotus

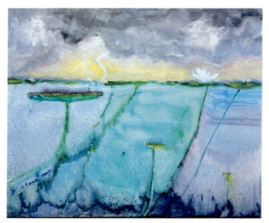

Awakening

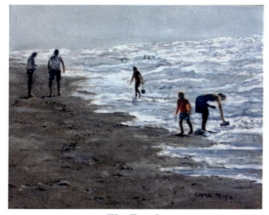

The Beach

FROM THE INSIDE OUT

Made in the USA
Columbia, SC
20 February 2021